Beyond Health

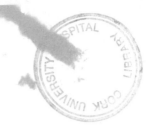

Beyond Health

Postmodernism and Embodiment

Nick J. Fox

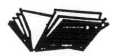

FREE ASSOCIATION BOOKS/LONDON/NEW YORK

i 14308095

First published in Great Britain by
Free Association Books
57 Warren Street, London W1P 5PA

© Nick J. Fox 1999

The right of Nick J. Fox to be identified as the author of this work has been
asserted by him in accordance with the Copyright, Designs and Patents Act 1988.

ISBN 1 85343 468 X hbk, 1 85343 469 8 pbk

A CIP catalogue record for this book is available from the British Library

Designed and produced for
Free Association Books by
Chase Production Services, Chadlington
Printed in the EU by J.W. Arrowsmith Ltd, Bristol

Contents

For Elisabeth,
and to the memory of
Gilles Deleuze and Felix Guattari

Preface

Looking down on the red landscape of South Australia from six miles up, I felt like the pilot of a spaceship over the surface of Mars or some other alien planet. I was so high that the shapes of the landscape had no perspective. Were those tiny dots bushes and scrub, or one hundred-foot-high gum trees? Were the geometrical shapes that seemed to divide the land man-made or some strange phenomenon of nature? Were the dried-out features ponds or vast lakes? Now I had fresh insight into the aboriginal people's paintings of their land, its awesome size and its character as a canvas patterned by intensities and differences. Those dreaming paintings were both of an external country and an inner landscape of events and places which together constitute a subjectivity, a sense-of-self.

I reread Chatwin's *The Songlines* before I left England, to think more about his reflections on nomadism in the context of aboriginal culture. As my plane carried me to Adelaide and I looked out of my window at the Australian continent, nomadic subjectivity seemed so much more possible than in the tiny crowded islands of Britain. Here – I knew – was a place where it would be easy to resist, to become, to move beyond whatever had been one's nature until now. And yet, both the landscape moving slowly beneath me, and my knowledge of aboriginal history since European colonization, reminded me of how hard it was to be a nomad, how many forces imposed themselves on a land's contours and an individual's life.

Nomadism is not restricted to the inhabitants of Australia, and this book is about the nomadic project for people with bodies, wherever they live. But it is not wholly a coincidence that this book was completed while in Australia, and I thank that country for the inspiration it provided. This book has been a long time in coming, and it is not quite what I had originally planned as the sequel to *Postmodernism, Sociology and Health* (Fox 1993a). It is a sequel, but it has a different objective, and a different audience. Whereas in my last book my effort was focused on a critique of sociology's modernism, here I am concerned with a very practical issue: embodiment.

Postmodernism is not – as many argue – a vapid, theoretical exercise in navel-gazing. At least as I conceive it, it is an ethical and political project, concerned with engagement with the world, on the side of resistance, and celebrating rather than bemoaning difference and otherness. Were this not the case, I would wish to have nothing to do with postmodern theory. This book uses postmodernism, but the emphasis is on the use, the practice. Think of it as a practical guide, not a book of theory.

Beyond health? It's a title that sums up for me the aspiration to escape, refuse and resist the conceptualization of embodiment by the institutions of disciplinary modernity, particularly modern medicine and the caring professions. I want to suggest that it is possible to have a non-essentialist yet becoming-body, not a being-body, not to be trammelled by notions of health and illness. I want to argue for a notion of embodiment so extensive that the notion of 'health' seems petty and narrow. Above all, I want to suggest that this is a project for everyone – individually *and* collectively, not some narrow academic treatise.

This book marks the first report of research I undertook concerning care. In 1997 I travelled to Thailand and Australia to do field-work on older adults' experiences as recipients of care. This research helped me to refine my understanding of the disciplinary and gift-like aspects of caring, and has been central to the nomadic theory of embodiment developed here. It was a wonderful experience to meet with all the older adults, some in residential homes in Australia, others in the back of beyond in hill villages in northern Thailand. I would like to take this opportunity to thank all the people I talked with during this field-work.

There are a huge number of people whom I should like to mention as contributing to my work over the past years as this book took shape. For getting me started on thinking about postmodernism: Helen Nicholson and Jane Naish; thanks also to Wendy Stainton Rogers who first suggested I look at Deleuze and Guattari's work. Elisabeth Galena and Sarah Long have been profoundly – though differently – significant in supplying spiritual nourishment. Thanks to Di Durie, Kim Campbell, Ruth Anne Reese and members of the *postmodern-christian* discussion group for general encouragement over the years to seek (and I believe, find) *rapprochement* between these two perspectives.

In Thailand, thanks to Sompong Chareonsuk, Linchong Pothiban, Sucharee Laorakpang, Duangruedee Lasuka, Nat Lukkhatai and countless other staff at the Faculty of Nursing, Chiang Mai University who enabled my visit and gave so much assistance in helping me interview older adults and translating. I was overwhelmed by the generosity and helpfulness of everyone I met in Chiang Mai, and special thanks are due to my friends Thongsouy (Air) Sitanon, Jariyaporn (Pui) Srisawang, Poorin and Jackarine for their welcome and affection.

In Australia, thanks to Julianne Cheek and David Gillham for hosting me at the University of South Australia, Adelaide, and to other staff there who facilitated my study leave and subsequent visits. At Flinders University, many thanks to my friends Jackie Morris, Jason Pudsie, Susie Duggin and Lisa Hancock for stimulating conversation and late nights out, also to Maria Zadoroznyj, John Coveney and members of the postmodernism discussion group. Thanks to Alan Petersen at Murdoch University and Ros Petersen for hospitality, and to Deborah Lupton at Charles Sturt University. Thanks to the staff at the residential homes I visited during field-work.

At the University of Sheffield, thanks to Nigel Mathers for constant encouragement and support for my research and writing, also to Richard Jenkins, Phil Levy and the WISDOM team for their general enthusiasm and stimulating company. Many thanks to Gillian Taberner for access to her data on the use of Ecstasy. Finally, a thank-you to David Stonestreet and the staff at Free Association Books.

Sheffield and Adelaide

Introduction:
The Promise of Postmodernism

There is an old joke about the person who, having lost their way, asks a local for directions to such and such a place. 'Ah, yes', replies the local, 'I know the place. But if I were going there, I wouldn't start from here.' While this quip works because it suggests an absurdity, there is actually an element of wisdom here. Some places are harder to get to from certain locations, while other routes are more straightforward. At the outset of this book, which looks *beyond* health, we can see two ways in which the joke is apposite to what follows.

First, it is actually hard to get to a position *beyond* health (at least in the way I am planning to get there) from the perspective of thinking about health in a traditional manner. And second, it is difficult to engage with postmodern social theory – this is the shorthand for the kinds of perspective I shall draw on in this book – when starting from the position of modernism.

The troubles which beset such travellers are exemplified in the comment in one recent text (the authorship of which perhaps should remain obscured) that 'postmodernism is really only an option for the healthy, not the sick'. It seemed 'obvious' to this authority, brought up in a modernist world-view, that the 'certainties of modern medicine' would be preferable to the complexities and problematizations of the world as seen by the post-modern theorist. The trouble with this kind of comment is that it is rather like asking a fish to appraise the merits of water as opposed to air: few would be able to grasp that their milieu could be anything other than the most desirable of all substances. Modernism is a pervasive medium which affects all the norms and values we have, and the way we see. Just as religious dogmatism prevented the recognition of the implications of scientific observations in the medieval era, today modernism has tainted all that it touches, making it hard for its acolytes to see differently.

1

But all is not gloom. Social theory is renowned for its critical character, and has valiantly refused on many occasions to accept the common-sense view of the world as a given. What is needed is the capacity to stand back, to question assumptions and be willing to try new ways of seeing. Anyone who has taken even a basic course in social science will know how threatening the theories of the social can be, whether they derive from Marxism, ethnomethodology or social constructionism. All may be rejected because they offend deeply held beliefs about the world, accreted over the years from a myriad of sources. Yet, while a commitment to modernism *is* the wrong place from which to start in an exploration of an alternative perspective, the sceptical modernist social theorist can try to avoid 'going native' in modernism. In particular, it may be possible to see new directions and complementaries, rather than inimical oppositions. With such an effort, I hope that the attempt to go 'beyond health' with which this book engages will be rewarding, even for those who remain embedded within modernism.

Let me unpack this issue of how we see health and illness a little, to set the tone for what follows. The ideas in this book are based on the proposition that health is not fundamentally a biological attribute. Similarly, it will argue that illness is not simply a biological deviation which – as far as is humanely possible – is to be addressed and resolved through the various technologies which medicine, nursing and therapy or complementary techniques have on offer. Up to that point, it is not saying anything particularly radical: most social scientists would acknowledge that health and illness are both natural and cultural. Health has economic, political and social ramifications, while illness is not equivalent to disease or pathology but depends upon social definition and individual experience (Kleinman 1988).

The real question, however, lies in the relation between nature and culture. Is the cultural component to health super-structural, build upon a foundational and ultimately determining biology (the 'realist' position)? Alternatively, is culture all, and nature an irrelevance (an extreme constructionism)? Or is it the case that culture and nature are more intricately associated, in ways which cannot be reduced to notions of base and superstructure, and require careful explication?

Mine is the last view. I do not accept the realist proposition that there is an absolute reality which is constituted around our biology. Neither shall I throw out the notion that biology is unimportant to the ways in which we think about health and illness, or can be 'transcended' by culture or by act of will: a kind of 'mind over matter' proposition. Instead, this book will suggest that this kind of dualism forces us to start thinking about these ideas of health and illness from the wrong place. Once we have set up the duality of culture/biology, we are led down a trail which sets up all sorts of new oppositions and dualities, including that of health/illness. We need to stand back from this kind of dichotomy, in which there is always a struggle for supremacy between one pole and another. It is the desire to overcome these oppositions which leads me away from modernist commitments and towards its critique: the body of theory which – perhaps inappropriately – is known as *post*modern. (The inappropriateness derives from the critical nature of postmodern theory. Postmodern social theory should be seen not as in *opposition* to modernism, but as a *commentary* upon it, a 'meta-text' which unsettles and chips away at modernist assumptions and hubris.)

The debate around a nature/culture duality is ultimately impoverished. It began way back with the nature or nurture debates over child behaviour and other issues in psychology including race, gender and intelligence (Rose 1989). The political correctness of the 1970s and thereafter (based on the perspective that all humans are born equal) enabled sociologists to claim a great victory over the biological determinists. But socio-biology has fought back with its arguments that behaviour is determined at the level of the species as well as the individual (Dawkins 1989). We are victims of our genes, and our sex and sexuality, our organizational behaviour and the ways we think about problems are consequences of our genetic make-up as well as our cultural background. More recently we have witnessed efforts by realist sociologists to embrace the biological, in the belief that such a *rapprochement* can save the discipline from the worst excesses of social constructionism and postmodern theory (Benton 1991).

Of course, what transpires from such activities is not a dissolution of the dualism but a reinvigoration of its division, but with a sociology which has strengthened itself against attack by incorporating part of its enemy's arsenal of arguments. We are expected to celebrate a sociology which can address issues rooted in the physiology of the organism such as emotions or pain (Williams and Bendelow 1998), while ignoring the fact that as a discipline, sociology excluded these elements from discussion in the first place because they did not sit comfortably within a subject which depended for its conceptual differentiation upon denial of the biological and an emphasis on the social!

The reason I am unimpressed by these antics is that they inadequately theorize the concepts of 'biology' and 'culture'. Biology is taken as a given rather than being subjected to scrutiny to understand the underpinning commitments of its disciplinary position; it is taken to be non-problematic, yet the level of naiveté about biological reasoning would never be accepted if it were a social science that were under the microscope. Functionalism is (almost) dead in cultural theory, yet biology is grounded in the explanatory power of a coupling of structure with function. Biology has told us there must be a functional reason for every characteristic of the living organism, with this extreme form of functionalism achieving its apogee in evolutionary theory. Are we really prepared to re-embrace this functionalist model of human behaviour, a model which can never be disproved because its twisted logic can impute an apparent purpose for virtually any behaviour?

Health is an arena in which the cultural and the natural are forced into juxtaposition. Like gender and ageing, the sub-discipline of social theory which addresses health must acknowledge the consequences of embodiment. But, as I shall show, this does not mean accepting the body as a given, nor the phenomena of birth, growth, death and disease as givens. To move *beyond* health will mean transforming how we think about virtually every aspect of our being, and a reconceptualization of how what have been traditionally called 'the biological' and 'the cultural' are to be understood. My intention is to rethink the categories and oppositions which depend upon the culture/nature dichotomy, and to see where that leads. Inevitably this amounts to a substantial project, which in effect requires a renewal of our notions of what it is to be human, or a living being for that matter. What are the concepts which we must deconstruct (and subsequently reconstruct)? We may list at least the following:

the body and embodiment
health and illness
time, growth and ageing
biology and the biological
sociology and the social
humanity and human *being*

In the remainder of this chapter, I want to set out the bare bones of this deconstruction. This means both setting the scene for the project and starting the critique of modernism which can help reinvent the notion of health. Most of the tools which will be used in this process derive from the post-structuralist or postmodern perspective. As the book pans out, I will use these tools as and when they are needed; in this introduction I shall sketch in a broader picture. My use of a register other than the dull prose of the modern will, I hope, *evoke* (Tyler 1986) in readers something of the mood of renewal and transformation which underpins this book. The allegorical figure which I have chosen for these opening pages is that of the *promise* (a concept with a postmodern pedigree: having been explored by Derrida (1987a) in his study of Poe's 'The Purloined Letter').

Three Promises

Promises are gifts. And when promises come to fruition (which all promises do, or they are not promises but empty words) it is doubly sweet because – despite the waiting and the anticipation – we have known all along, we have trusted and been certain that they would be fulfilled. The trip to the zoo, the first night of wedded passion, the Promised Land of the Israelites, feel so good when finally happening, because they were presaged in the promise. Moses would not have been so willing to wander for years in the desert (and die before he arrived) were the Promised Land to have been the Land That Could Be Yours One Day or the Land I Might Give You If You're Good. The Promised Land was already a gift, which could not be taken away: the Israelites could trust God not to renege; they were empowered, knowing that his love was unconditional, that however badly they behaved, one day the gift would be in their hands.

Promises thus stand in place of that which is promised: they are a sign of what is to be given. English banknotes carry a promise from the British Government that, on demand, it will 'pay the bearer the sum of such-and-such'. In theory at least, we could exchange these promissory notes for 'real money', although the latter would in turn be a further *signifier* (as opposed to the referent) of the wealth of the nation which backs the currency. Like the Promised Land, banknote promises are special because of the trust, and the faith, which sustain them; they are built on relationship, and without relationship they are meaningless (as is witnessed when currencies collapse). This relationship of trust empowers, it allows us to travel in time, to look forward (in both senses) to a future fulfilment, and be confident of a continuity of relationship. As the root of the word *promise* reminds us, they 'go before' what is to come, they are the guarantor of what has already been given, but is not yet here and now.

Promises are not coercive, their recipients can choose whether to take up the promised gift or not. We can leave our banknotes under the bed, to use when we wish. That is why promises are such special gifts – they are gifts given without expectation of reciprocity. They offer a future, but do not force it down our throat, demanding we be grateful. Promises free us, make new possibilities available; they are the victory of life over death, a becoming-other in place of stagnation. They are inscribed in letters of love.

It is particularly appropriate to speak of the promise of postmodernism, for the ethics and politics of this position (at least as I shall explore them) are about 'becoming' rather than being, about diversification and multiplicity, about relationship and giving. Within this ethos, it is inappropriate to enter into rancorous debate about the advantages of 'modern' or 'postmodern' social theory; debates which substitute fear and misunderstanding for exploration, dialogue and engagement. The promise of postmodernism lies in its emphasis on openness, diversity and freedom.

The first promise of postmodernism is the promise to open up the discourses which fabricate our bodies and our health and illness. The discourses of medicine and its collaborators in the modernist human sciences seek to territorialize us as 'organisms' – *bodies-with-organs* (Deleuze and Guattari 1984), doomed to face the ministrations of these disciplines – to 'health', 'beauty' to a 'full and active life', to patience in the face of the failure of senses and memory, to accept, to *be*, never again to become other. Against these formulations, we are now rediscovering that our embodiment is provisional, we are cyber-bodies, already stretching the limits of our humanity, free to roam, to make ourselves other. So we may think not of a health fabricated by the body-with-organs, but of *arché-health*, a 'health' which is much more than 'health', which cannot be spoken because to speak it would inscribe it, and of *nomads,* subjectivities resisting and refusing discourse, not patients but impatients. (Both these concepts will be fully explored in the text which follows.)

The disciplines of the self are so seductive: they permeate the way we act, what we eat, how we regulate our behaviour, how and to whom we make love (Foucault 1986). Even the care we offer each other is territorialized, as the rationality of the modernist market place encroaches even into the privatized spaces where emotion and love are hidden away. Relationships are based on reciprocity: caring *about* someone becomes caring *for* someone (Gardner 1992). Care is transformed into a *vigil* (Fox 1995a) through the activities of theorists (including social theorists) which has the power to territorialize those who care and those who receive it, from cradle to grave.

The second promise of postmodernism is that – despite this disciplining work of the academy and of practitioners of health and care – it is possible to engage with those we encounter in those environments in ways which are not disciplinary, and which indeed challenge discipline. Such engagements are not about 'empowering', because what is involved is not *power* at all, but love and the *gift*. It is the antidote to academic or clinical *hubris,* a recognition that we cannot disengage from the world and our lives through the construction of a realm of the academic or the clinic – or that if we do try to disengage, that the tragic irony of this will face each of us when we are confronted by our mortality and our humanness. This promise of postmodernism is a hard one. It reminds us of the context of all our energetic actions, that we are human and must die, and that those we love will die and be gone one day too.

Yet our humanness is not tragic, it is a reason to celebrate. The ethics and politics of postmodernism are based in difference, in acknowledging diversity, that the world and its inhabitants do not fit into neat academic categories. So as we grieve for our finitude, we delight in our human diversity. We are no longer theorists separated from those we study, or practitioners distanced from our patients or clients (relationships of the kind that Cixous (1986) called the *proper*), but participants, sharing and giving of ourselves.

The final promise of postmodernism is that we can start this right away, and that it is for all of us: social or cultural theorist, practitioner, parent, lover. It is that it is possible to engage with others in ways which will open up possibilities, not close down the way people think or behave. We can give of ourselves without seeking reciprocity (indeed, we give in this way all the time and never know it). That we can love and care, not wanting that the other be *like* something, but that the other is other. That we can be nomadologists (Deleuze and Guattari 1988), creating new spaces to inhabit whatever we do, with whomever we engage.

Two Icons: the Detective and the Nomad

The Post-Enlightenment or modern period celebrates rationality. Foucault (1970) identified this period with the development of the modern scientific disciplines of labour, life and language (economics, biology and philology) and the human 'sciences' which built on them (sociology, psychology and the study of literature and myth). Modernity and modernism are thought of as coinciding with philosophical commitments to truth, rationalism and rationalization, with progress. the belief that scientific analysis is the means by which the world will come to be known, and with humanism: the centring of the human subject as the wellspring of knowledge and good.

The ethos of modernism is typified in the consulting detective Sherlock Holmes, complete with fawning public in the shape of Watson, always ready to be astounded by the latest discovery. The icon of the postmodern is not western at all; it is far from that Victorian rationalist with his comfortable consulting rooms and servant/surrogate mother, Mrs Hudson. It is the *nomad*.

The nomad does not put down roots, or manipulate her environment to suit her needs and wishes. She does not seek control; she takes what is on offer, assimilates it, and moves on. She is at war with the forces which would territorialize her, the rationalism which values the stable, the static and the instrumentalism of matching actions to goals (Deleuze and

Guattari 1988: 380). Civilization, norms, taste, social distinctions mean nothing to her: she is at one with her environment, yet never part of it. She is a warrior without a strategy (ibid.: 353, Plant 1993).

The association of postmodernism, whether sceptical or affirmative (Rosenau 1992) with fragmentation, multivocality, radical doubt over meta-narratives, epistemological relativism and anti-essentialism generates this nomad. We can see the nomadism of postmodernism in the texts of various writers including Derrida, Foucault, Lyotard, Deleuze and Guattari, Cixous and others. The account which is the most explicit derives from Deleuze and Guattari, and it is worth briefly acknowledging the components of this perspective (which are fully developed in chapter 5).

Deleuze and Guattari start their journey towards the nomad with their analysis of embodiment. For them, the body is not the physical biological entity of biomedicine (they call this 'the organism'). Rather the body is a psychic or philosophical surface which is imprinted by the forces of the social (Deleuze and Guattari 1984: 9ff). From the moment of birth – perhaps even before – this body or *Body-without-Organs (BwO)* is inscribed by its interaction with the world. The need for nourishment, for warmth and comfort, the disciplining of the nursery and the schoolroom, the gendering and sexualization of adolescence, the routines of work and the growth and disillusionment of ageing all inscribe the BwO. Yet the BwO is not passive, it is at the same time as it is inscribed, both the author of inscription and an affirmation of potential.

For Deleuze and Guattari, there is a continual struggle in the realm of the social between *smooth* and *striated* spaces (Deleuze and Guattari 1988: 370–1). Striated space is the consequence of acts of power, which homogenize the environment around particular organizing principles. Smooth spaces are heterogeneous, in which difference reigns. There are no channels or connections between points: in every direction the perspective is similarly amorphous. The Body-without-Organs may, through its inscription with the forces of the social (what could traditionally be imagined as 'socialization') come to move in striated space.

Deleuze and Guattari use the analogy of a game of chess (ibid.: 353), in which each piece has moves proper to itself, and cannot inhabit the entire field of struggle. But it is also possible for the BwO to break free from striation (through the affirmation of its potential to *be other*, and with the assistance of others) and move into smooth space. Deleuze and Guattari compare smooth space with the game of Go, in which pieces are functionally undifferentiated, and achieve their objectives by *territorializing* and *deterritorializing* space (ibid.). Go pieces are nomadic, while chess pieces are agents of a State apparatus, organized according to rules and hierarchy.

The human body is continually implicated in the territorializing of smooth space and the deterritorializing of striated spaces. One such territorialization is the construction of a biomedical version of the body: the *organism*. The organism is the striation of the BwO, which organizes, folds, delimits, names the un-named. Because its striation is organized in principles of biology and pathology, it is the organism 'from which doctors benefit, and on which they base their power' (ibid.: 159). The smooth space of the BwO becomes the organism through the persistent inscription of biology and medical science. The *nomad* is both the opponent of the organism, and the outcome of a deterritorializing of the organism. The nomadic BwO wanders in a field in which biology has not constructed a map: there are no landmarks, and no familiar paths.

The organism is a creation of culture, it is a historical outcome of civilization. Foucault's dramatic illustration of the contested character of the human body in the opening pages of *The Birth of the Clinic* (1976: ix-xii), describes the great changes between the eighteenth and nineteenth centuries in how those who explored the interior of the body saw. Something which at one point in history was made visible by power/knowledge in one way, would appear quite differently under a different regime of knowledge, even when the observers claimed a continuity of discipline (in this case, anatomy). New disciplines within medical science: physiology, embryology, immunology, have since vied to fabricate the body authentically, to speak the truth about it. More recently, psychology and sociology have had an impact, with some of their concepts incorporated in medical discourse, as a biopsychosocial model of medicine transforms the early biomedical body (Armstrong 1987). New medical technologies such as cloning and gene therapy and manipulation challenge our sense of what it means to be human.

Yet there is no 'truth' out there concerning the way the body really is. We may have sense data from that materiality, but these data are organized by the striations of the social. Similarly, every datum from the internal world of sensation and pain is refracted through the lens of the social as we process it into 'experience' of our bodies and ourselves. Such experiences come to have a life of their own, and we lose sight of their origins in the territorialization of the BwO. Only through deterritorializing striated space may we be freed to wander like the nomad.

In this way, postmodernism challenges the facticity of the human body as constituted in biology, psychology and modernist social theory. Foucault's various genealogies of power, knowledge and the disciplining of the body (1976, 1979, 1984, 1986) describe the inscription of this body by discourse, including those on health and illness. The BwO is a bodily, affective *subjectivity*, fabricated in 'the complex interplay of highly constructed social and symbolic forces ... the body is a play of forces, a surface of intensities' (Braidotti 1993: 44).

I mentioned earlier the process of growing old as part of the territorial-izing of the BwO. Ageing is not only a physical phenomenon, it is a complex interplay of cellular and organic degeneration, psychology, affec-tivity and the micropolitics of the social and the cultural. In chapter 2, I shall look at how time territorializes the BwO of the older adult, cutting across the patternings of subjectivity which have previously constituted the person's sense-of-self. Now she responds in ways 'proper' to her age, accepting limitations and generating cognitions, emotions and patterns of behaviour to inform and pad out this new subjectivity. Her age may be read (and mis-read) by others in demeanour and in interaction, reinforcing or refining the subject. The subject adopts new bodily strategies (self-care, risk reduction or perhaps abandonment), through which she in turn is reconstituted and reread.

It is in such explorations that we find the first promise of postmod-ernism, to open up new possibilities for how we understand bodies, health and illness. Nomadology challenges the socialization of age, suggesting possibilities for a smoothing out of the striations, a renewal or a transfor-mation. More broadly, it establishes the basis for the radically different conception of human potential which I call *arché-health* (Fox 1993a).

Arché-health

Arché-health is not a concept in opposition or antagonistic to that of health. Rather it is the condition of possibility for health or illness. It is the smoothing out of the striations which enable us variously to speak of health and illness. Biology, medicine, psychology, sociology all have their favourite definitions of health, and my documenting of these (Fox 1993a: 138) will stand repetition. Traditionally, health was defined simply as an absence of illness, but the World Health Organization (WHO 1985) sought a more holistic (if vacuous) definition, and considers health to be the state of 'complete physical, mental and social well-being'. From an anthropological perspective, Wright (1982) sees health as 'what it is to function as a human' with illness defined as circumstances of a failure to function which continues to be seen as human. Canguilhem (1989) defines health and illness as positive and negative biological values. Illness is a 'notion of increasing dependency' for de Swaan (1990: 220), and Sedgewick identified illnesses as socially constructed definitions of natural circumstances which precipitate death or a failure to function according to certain values (1982: 30).

All these definitions (medical and sociological) are striations or territorializations: they act on the BwO, constituting it in particular ways. As such, they are political, acts of power which seek *mastery*, and constitutive of subjectivity and of embodiment. The postmodern promise is the substitution of this will to mastery with an *affirmation of potential* (Massumi 1992: 174) or commitment to otherness. As such it comprises an ethics and an attitude of resistance to power. Nomadology is deeply political.

The need for such an ethics and politics can be demonstrated by a reading of the work of Oliver Sacks (1991, 1995), who has documented the refusals and rejections of medicalizing definitions of health and illness among his patients. A woman in her eighties who had contracted tertiary syphilis liked her pathology, because it made her feel 'frisky'. An artist who lost his colour sight refused a chance to restore it, having developed a way of seeing and creating in monochrome. The 'awakening' of people treated with L-Dopa for their Parkinsonism was in many cases a shattering and highly distressing experience. How many people are persuaded into 'cures' which cut across their subjectivity, inscribing a new medical identity – with no acknowledgement of their 'right' to otherness?

So a responsibility to otherness, in relation to issues of 'health' and 'illness', will suggest a radically different conception of human potential, and this is what is meant by *arché-health*. *Arché-health* is a becoming, a deterritorializing of the BwO, a resistance to discourse, a generosity towards otherness, a nomadic subjectivity. It is not intended to suggest a natural, essential or in any way prior kind of health, upon which the other healths are superimposed. It is not supposed to be a rival concept, indeed the reason for using this rather strange term is its homage to Derrida's (1976: 56) notion of *arché-writing*, which is not writing but that which supplied the possibility of writing, that is, the system of difference upon which language is based: *différance* – that which differs and is deferred. Similarly, *arché-health*:

- is the *becoming* of the organism which made it possible for the first time to speak of health or illness.
- is present, in the sense that a trace of it is carried, in every discourse on health, however and with whatever *logos* that discourse has constituted itself.
- can never become the object of scientific investigation, without falling back into discourse on health/illness. It is not the outcome of deconstruction of these discourses, it *is* deconstruction: difference and becoming.
- is multiple in its effects. As difference, it is meaningless to speak of its unity or its division.

Every BwO has an *arché-health*, which is its *becoming other*. Whereas health and illness territorialize the BwO by their discourses, *arché-health* is the refusal and resistance to this discourse. Your, or my, *arché-health* may be more or less developed, depending how territorialized our subjectivities are by the discourses of medicine and the social sciences. It is the path towards the BwO, one which is a life-long journey:

> You never reach the Body-without-Organs, you can't reach it, you are forever attaining it, it is a limit. ... But you're already on it, scurrying like a vermin, groping like a blind person, or running like a lunatic: desert travels and nomad of the steppes. On it we sleep, live our waking lives, fight – fight and are fought – seek our place, experience untold happiness and fabulous defeats: on it we penetrate and are penetrated: on it we love. (Deleuze and Guattari 1988: 150)

The ethics and politics of *arché-health* are deconstructive, reminding us to ask hard questions of the modernist disciplines which inscribe us into subjectivity through their conceptions of, and preoccupations with, 'health' and 'illness'.

The Gift and the Proper

Imagine on one hand the people in our lives who say, '... be this ... do this for me ... I want you to be like this ...'. Their discourses reflect their desire (which is a lack or a wish) for you to be like them, to take on an identity which supports their own sense-of-self: Such talk *territorializes* the BwO, patterning it with a subjectivity which creates it in the image of that lack or wish.

On the other hand there is the person who says, '... here's some space for you ... go for it ... get on with it ... I trust and have confidence in you ... take my generosity of spirit'. This kind of engagement is a *gift* which enables, opens up new possibilities, allows the BwO to differentiate, to *deterritorialize* for a moment, to establish a nomad subjectivity, to resist.

Which kind of person are you? If you are an academic or a member of the practical professions concerned with health and care – like it or not – it's likely that you are the first kind, although educators and professionals who are 'facilitative' in their practice may have broken with such disciplinary approaches. Modernism's *will to mastery* is Sherlock Holmes at work again, always categorizing, diagnosing, analyzing, testing hypotheses, developing theory. Consequently it is very hard to deterritorialize our

BwOs from the discourses which have grown up in medicine, nursing and the social sciences. We need all the help we can get.

I suggested earlier, following White (1991), that the ethics and politics of postmodernism replace the commitment to mastery and action with a commitment to otherness and difference. In writing of a *gift*, this term is used advisedly, recalling my remarks concerning promises, and drawing on the recent work of Derrida (1992) and the feminist post-structuralist Cixous (1986). Cixous opposes *gift* relationships to what she sees as the masculine realm of the *proper* (property, possession, propriety), of possessive desire based in a wish and a lack, identity and dominance (Cixous 1986, Moi 1985). If we were concerned with an ethical engagement with other people – be they lovers, children, clients, students or colleagues, then the characteristics of such gift relationships would seem particularly appropriate as the basis for our relationships.

In an effort to deconstruct earlier notions of gifts based in reciprocity (Mauss 1990), Derrida (1992) speaks of the true gift as that which one does not realize one is giving. It is the gift which has the capacity to deterritorialize, to create smooth space. Maussian gifts by contrast, territorialize and create striation where formerly there was smoothness, because of the rules of reciprocity they impose at the moment of their giving. Gifts like these reflect *proper* relationships, and in the realm of the *proper*, a gift is thus threatening because it establishes an inequality, a difference, an imbalance in power. The act of giving becomes an act of aggression, an exposure of the other (Moi 1985: 112). Gifts may also serve other purposes, as the commentary on the hypocritical giving of the Pharisees in the Christian New Testament reminds us: their 'gifts' were outward shows of godliness, intended to define their own superiority, and perhaps to store up credit for the after-life. In contrast, the *gift* is not given with any expectation of reciprocity; in the realm of the *gift*, those who give do not expect gratefulness or even an acknowledgement of their effort.

The force and value of this distinction between the *gift* and the *proper* (between the Derridean and the Maussian gift) rest in the possibility that things could be different. It offers the potential for an ethics and politics of engagement based on a celebration of difference, not of identity (Haber 1994). The *proper* is a possessive relationship, constantly requiring of its object that it behaves in certain ways, that it is defined (as 'patient', 'student', 'sociology'), and repeats the patterns of those who have been the objects of its discourse previously. Substituting *gift* relationships changes everything: we engage with others now as others, not as those with whom we might wish to identify. Definition is replaced with metaphor and allusion, analysis and theory with poetics and expression, professional care by love and the celebration of difference.

We must not underestimate the impact (and difficulty) of replacing the *proper* in the disciplines of care and the academy. Substituting such relations with those based on *gifts* is about replacing a modernist responsibility to act with a responsibility to otherness (White 1991). White suggests that this means adopting what he describes as a mood of 'grieving delight'. One grieves for human finitude, but delights and celebrates difference (Fox 1993a: 130). Grief sensitizes us to injustice, while delight deepens our concern with celebrating difference in our humanity.

This takes us back to *arché-health,* which is about this dual engagement with the other. Whether as a member of a care profession or as an academic, we are to be guided by a responsibility to otherness which has as its objective the facilitation of becoming, of *arché-health. Arché-health* is possible only by the deterritorialization of the BwO, resisting its inscription of the relations of the *proper.* I will develop these ideas much more fully in chapter 3.

Nomadology for Beginners

To return to Sherlock Holmes and the nomad. Holmes uses language and the signs by which he makes sense of 'reality' in the same way a physician diagnoses diseases from signs and symptoms, to deduce what occurred at a location. Every clue 'speaks' to him of what is absent, drawing upon a regime of truth based in assumptions about the world. ('When you have eliminated the impossible, whatever remains, however improbable, must be the truth.') He is the modernist *par excellence,* persuading himself and us that his fabrications are synonymous with reality – even when reality is very strange.

The nomad (although there are no nomads, only nomadism and nomadic existence – it is a mood or an ethos, not a state of being) is like Holmes in one way, in that she is continually slipping into the detective's way of thinking, mistaking her constructions of reality for truth. She is attracted by discourses which offer certainty, she is at war with her own longing for a fixed point. Yet the medium of language which enslaves is also the medium of resistance to discourse. Achieving nomadism (and in realizing that it is never finally achieved), means contesting the patternings of subjectivity which discourses inscribe on the BwO, and the medium of this contestation is language. Cixous talks about the power of language:

A feminine text cannot fail to be more than subversive. It is volcanic, as it is written it brings about an upheaval of the old property crust, carrier of masculine investments, there's no other way ... it's in order to smash everything, to shatter the framework of institutions, to blow up the law, to break up the 'truth' with laughter. (Cixous 1990: 326)

Similarly, Deleuze and Guattari see writing as a way of 'deterritorializing', of breaking free from discourse, refusing to follow a single chain of meaning (1988: 7–9). Their own writing, in particular their book *A Thousand Plateaus* (Deleuze and Guattari 1988), is intended to deterritorialize their readers, to offer new possibilities and new subjectivities. It is also about living in the here and now, not in the pasts and futures dreamed up in discourse (Braidotti 1993: 44).

We can see just such a deterritorialization in the virtualization of 'reality' in the new cyber-culture. In May 1995, I took part in a plenary discussion at the *Virtual Futures* conference with the two performance artists Stellarc and Orlan, to talk about their work and the ethics associated with it. Stellarc has begun to explore the philosophical challenges of the cyborg (part-human, part-machine) in a series of performances, including the construction of an artificial third arm, and the control of this and other parts of his body by strangers via the Internet. Orlan's performance art entails changing her appearance through plastic surgery – some of which is conventional, while the use of cheek inserts to create bumps on her temples challenges norms of human physiognomy and beauty. What Stellarc and Orlan have in common is a questioning of the limits of the body, and of what it means to be human and to live in relationship with other 'humans'. They are interested, as are the cyberpunk writers, in developing the post-human, who is free from the constraints of the body. William Gibson writes of a future in which humans are downloaded into computers, and carry on a non-corporeal existence in cyberspace: we are challenged to reflect on our relations with such 'constructs', and on their humanity (Bukatman 1993). Within cyber-culture, there is also a new eclectic spirituality which challenges the limitations of realist philosophy and scientific secularism (Rushkoff 1994). The implications for the kind of postmodern nomadology which I have been exploring are – I hope – clear: technology, literature and art, and cyber-spirituality are variously testing the limits of embodied humanity, as constituted in the traditional discourses of the body.

But as I conclude these introductory remarks, I want to turn back to the promise of postmodernism for those involved intimately with health and illness: 'patients' and their carers. Exploring care and the relationships between carers and those who receive care, I have been struck by the extent to which *proper* relations impinge on an area which – intuitively – one might expect to reflect the *gift* (Fox 1995a, 1995b). When I come, in chapter 2, to describe my research on older adults' experiences of care, I will document the territorializing effects of dependency and physical limitation. The ethics and politics of a commitment to difference and nomadism must involve a replacement of the *proper* by the *gift* in caring and healing relationships. But if this is easy to say, then it seems that it is far harder in practice: there are two issues here. First, it requires an overturning of the disciplinary bases of caring professions, and all that goes with professionalization: status, power and a differentiation from those who are cared for. Second, there is a need for a new way of thinking about humanity and the way we understand our lives and deaths.

The final promise of postmodernism addresses these two challenges. Generosity, trust, love, affirmation, confidence in the other supply the basis for an opportunity – here and now – to be other, not more of the same. The rest of this book will be about the pursuit of the nomadic moment in which subjectivity is freed, and this nomad subject *becomes*. In that moment we will see how it is possible to be human.

Structure of the Book

In this introduction I have painted broad brush-strokes to illuminate my project, and have glossed many important ideas. In the chapters which follow, these ideas will be amplified and developed. The book divides into three sections, each of which is preceded by a brief summary, and an exegesis of the main theoretical concepts developed in the following pages. The first section addresses issues of power and control, and the way in which 'health' and 'illness' contribute to our subjectivity and sense of our selves. In the second part, a perspective on how it is possible to resist power is developed, and in the final section, I suggest ways to apply this position as part of a project of transformation or becoming.

Chapters 1, 2 and 3 explore the forces operating in health settings from a range of postmodern theoretical positions. In the first of these chapters, I look at how professionals 'frame' their encounters with patients in such a way to silence alternative readings, using theoretical perspectives from Derrida's analysis of the frame and Lyotard's notion of the 'differend'. Chapter 2 introduces research data on caring settings, to show how space and time are constitutive of a modernist and limiting notion of health. Chapter 3 is a pivotal exploration of caring, which sets the scene for the rest of the book. It suggests a dual character for care, as both a disciplinary project which constrains and as a potentially enabling and transforming interaction which opens up possibilities for those who are its recipients.

Having identified the controlling character of health care organization, the second section addresses the crucial issue of how to conceptualize resistance to control within a non-essentialist framework. Foucault's work has been highly influential in the sociology of health, yet it fails to explain how actors may resist power. Chapter 4 analyses Foucault's model, and argues that something more is required from a post-structuralist account of human action. The following chapter suggests such an alternative, outlining the three principles in Deleuze and Guattari's work of relevance here: the *Body-without-Organs*, *territorialization* and *nomadology*. Each is considered in relation to examples from health and care, and connections made with other theorists including Derrida and Haraway. The outcome is an understanding of a non-essentialist yet resisting subjectivity.

The last section of the book turns from theory to practice, to consider how this model of a resisting subject can be applied to suggest ways in which it is possible to 'become other'. Chapter 6 puts the theoretical work of the previous chapter to work, in a major analysis of an issue in health and care: risk and risk-taking – at work, and among users of Ecstasy. It is argued that notions of risk disguise active choice-making by human beings, and that subjectivity is an on-going project of becoming-other which amounts to *arché-health*. The following chapter looks at postmodern positions on knowledge in the research setting, and challenges the 'taken-for-granted' nature of the entities to be studied. I address the politics of research, and argue for a reflective approach, and a political commitment which challenges researcher/researched dichotomies. Action research and reflective research approaches are explored as possibilities for a postmodern research process. In chapter 8, I focus on the problems, possibilities and dangers associated with nomadism and becoming, and consider what a nomadic approach to living means generally, and specifically in settings of health and social care. In accordance with an emphasis upon reflexivity, the concluding pages of the book include some thoughts on the lived experience of the author and nomadology.

Part 1
FORCE

Introduction

If it were easy to move *beyond* health, then it would be something commonplace, a frequent event of little note. There would be no need for a book about it; more importantly, there would be no need to exert ourselves: we could accept that health/illness is all there is, however unattractive that prospect. In one respect we all continually move beyond health (or beyond illness) as our lives unfold. However we are also being continually drawn back to health/illness. By which I mean that we are continually returning to a way of being, a way of thinking about being, which is constraining and limiting.

Bodies are material, or at least, there is something there that is material. But this materiality cannot be known directly: the materiality of bodies and their states of being (called, amongst other things, 'health' and 'illness') are mediated through being known and 'make sense of', not at the level of the material, but at the level of the concept. To use a piece of postmodern jargon: knowledge of the referent (the materiality) is deferred by the intervention of the signification (the concept) used to give sense to the referent (Derrida 1976: 50). And this deferral is indefinite; there is never a moment in which the signification becomes transparent, when we can know what is beyond or behind the sign.

So moving *beyond health* cannot mean something transcendental, in the sense of something metaphysical or outside of the systems of signs which give us sense of the world. It does not mean getting to a more 'real' idea of the body, stripping away the falseness of language to reveal what is underneath. Rather, it means a breaking-free from a straightjacket: the limitations which the narrow concepts of 'health' and 'illness' impose. To pick up an idea from the introductory chapter, it is a promise of what *could* be. The glimpses of this promise are encouraging, yet the inevitable falling-back into traditional health/illness seems disheartening. How can

21

we make the necessary break which is needed? How can we substitute *arché-health* for these limiting states?

In management theory, the ideas of Kurt Lewin have been used to formulate a way of understanding systems dynamically (and as a tool for change) known as 'force-field analysis' (Lewin 1948). This simple model suggests that the equilibrium position of a system – a mental state, a family unit or an organizational system – is not a system at rest, but one in which dynamic opposing forces are at work. The current position is a consequence of balanced *driving* and *restraining* forces. Increase the former or decrease the latter, and the system moves to a new rest position. Keep altering one or other force, and the system will oscillate. Enhancing the power of those seeking change, or reducing the power which is holding the system back can change organization.

Add a further element, the notion of a feedback loop, and you gain subtlety. Negative feedback will tend to sustain driving and restraining forces in balance. A simple example is a thermostatically controlled device, which balances the cooling effects of the environment and the heating effects of a power source (or the converse, in an air conditioner or refrigerator), to sustain a constant ambient temperature. Positive feedback, on the other hand, pushes a system further and further from balance, increasing driving forces or decreasing restraining forces incrementally. Positive feedback drives chaotic or catastrophic systems, which become increasingly unstable and finally uncontrollable, like nuclear fission going 'critical'.

Imagine a force field such as this determining our current sense of 'health' and 'illness' (a complex which I shall refer to simply as health: health implies illness and vice versa, one cannot exist without the other). Despite driving forces which seek to break free from the limits of 'health', there are strong restraining forces at work. Negative feedback (a control mechanism such as a thermostat) ensures that whenever something beyond is glimpsed, the restraining forces strengthen, and we fall back on to the earlier sense of health. What is needed is a concerted push, something to increase the driving forces and then increase again. We need a positive feedback loop which will enable us to go critical.

There are two ways of achieving this. One is to increase the driving forces. The other, and the one which is often used in management, is to disable or reduce the restraining forces. Perhaps both are needed, and in this book I shall certainly consider both approaches. In the next chapters I shall consider the restraining forces and how they work. Then in part 2, I shall look at the driving forces, the forces resisting control. But before I begin, I need to make one thing very clear.

For all intents and purposes, bodies and their health/illness come into being only in the moment of signification. Prior to this moment, they are unknowable, even though they exist. From this, it follows that we can trace the shape of embodiment through the register of the signifier. In the analogy of the force field, embodiment is a consequence of the equilibrium between the driving forces and the restraining forces, the control and the resistance to control.

To go beyond health thus cannot simply mean shifting the balance a little. That would amount to no more than a resignification, a new conceptualization of health. In the introductory chapter we saw just this: the 57 varieties of 'health' defined by anyone and everyone. What I mean when I talk about going 'beyond health' is something other than merely creating a new definition. It has to be about abolishing the oppositions. More precisely, it is about deconstructing the register of signification altogether. *Arché-health* must stand outside this register: in the *system of difference* which made signification possible in the first place (Derrida 1976: 56). What is beyond health is a new figure of embodiment, constituted not from an endlessly deferring signification, but from difference itself, otherness, becoming.

1
Framing Health

From my study window, I can see the city of Sheffield spreading out across the valleys and hills upon which it is built. On the horizon I see the outlines of houses set against a sky tinged pink as afternoon shades into evening. The trees in my neighbours' gardens demarcate the view to the east. On the west, the houses recede in perspective, leading my eye toward the skyline. These elements of the view frame my outlook, as does the window itself.

Our perspectives on the world are never free of a frame. Even on the top of a hill with panoramic views, our eye sockets or our camera lenses frame what we see. The difference between a good and a poor photograph will depend in part on how it is framed: what is in the picture and what has been cropped. The job of the picture editor on a newspaper is to frame the pictures to maximize their impact. Framed with an appropriate caption, a close-up of a footballer shooting may be more evocative than one which shows player, ball and goal mouth.

Framing does not simply involve the sense organ and its biological limits. Psychology has demonstrated that perception is an active process, entailing more than simply gathering sense data (Gregory 1990). It requires interpretation of that data: we have to learn to see or hear, to distinguish the important from the irrelevant (signal from noise), to organize and seek familiar patterns in these data, to respond cognitively or emotionally to the data based on past experience or association. We can be fooled by these frames: a stage set designed to appear to possess normal perspective may in fact be cunningly distorted so that the unexpected occurs when an actor crosses. Within the frame of the set, the impossible can appear to happen.

Learning is also based on framing. 'Knowledge' is more than mere data, it derives from various manipulations. Data may be ordered, processed, patterned, distilled or trawled for key points, distorted, or whatever. What comes out of this is no longer 'pure': it has undergone a series of framings which – within a particular context – give it meaning, and potentially the right to be called 'knowledge' or 'truth'. Different disciplines (say psychology and sociology), or different theoretical perspectives (fundamentalist Christianity and evolution, for instance) may interpret the same data in quite different ways, selecting, excluding and perhaps mangling them to make them fit.

Here is a key insight: frames have the important property that they set limits which *exclude*, and by this exclusion enable us to fix on what is in the picture. As we have seen, framing is not limited to sense data: it is implicated in various cognitive activities including the strange activity of thinking, of 'the mind's eye' in which we can conceive, reflect, construct and deconstruct whatever we will. Thought is framed by experience, imagination, memory, affectivity and by the capacity for symbolic representation which humans (and perhaps other species) develop at an early age. Like my window frame or the horizon, these frames restrict, and yet, paradoxically, make sense and knowledge possible.

Although it may be argued that frames are necessary to help make sense of the world, they have a profound disadvantage. Some years back I attended a national exhibition of prize-winning children's art. Why, I wondered, was there such a difference between the paintings done by young children and those done by their older brothers and sisters? Those painted by the primary school children were vibrant, full of life and colour, powerful and imaginative. In comparison, the pictures done by 13- and 14-year-olds were mannered, derivative and lacking in any sense of creativity. I guessed that the older children were being taught established styles, and the mini-Picassos or para-Van Goghs which they produced possessed some technical expertise which the judges rewarded, but which were devoid of the raw creativity I had seen in the youngsters' work. In learning to imitate, framing their work in the traditions of art history, they had lost or become detached from the flair, motivation and powerful visions that had inspired them before they learnt method and technique.

Frames give us sense, they make meaning possible. But they also destroy, setting limits which exclude the chaotic and the unacceptable. As such, they are at the heart of culture and 'civilization'. We may value the achievements of a society framed by certain values, but we can see too the genocide (now reframed as 'ethnic cleansing') which killed off so many in the twentieth century because they did not fit within a frame. Frames limit what it is possible to think or see or believe, which is how and why they work. Thus, they are implicated in power and control. Resisting power may require us to recognize, question and reject the frame and its act of exclusion.

Texts, Frames and Differends

Deconstruction is an approach which is often seen as synonymous with post-structuralism and postmodern theory. It was developed – or given a name – by Derrida (1976: 49), to explore the workings of power in the textual construction of the social world. While the term has sometimes been used almost generically as a synonym for social analysis, this is to dilute deconstruction's focus on textuality and the strategies by which readings of situations are privileged through, and in the service of, power. In general, it works by overturning these privileged readings, examining the way the world would look if the opposing view were to be dominant. As such, it is potentially both anti-authoritarian and a tool for resistance (Critchley 1992, Rosenau 1992). Deconstruction has been applied in social theory to reveal the unspoken assumptions behind claims to 'truth' (Fox 1991, 1993a, Game 1991), and is of particular use in exploring how particular perspectives come to dominance, and what happens in situations where interpretations of reality are contested.

It should not be thought of as a method or methodology. It is more appropriate to think of deconstruction as a perspective, a mood, even a political position committed on the side of resistance, transformation and regeneration. The different approaches used in this book may all be seen as deconstructive, and in this chapter I develop three of these: the post-structuralist conception of *intertextuality* (Barthes 1977); Derrida's (1987b) analysis of the *frame* or boundary as the place at which power acts; and Lyotard's (1988) notion of the *differend*. The intention is both to illustrate the use of deconstructive approaches, and to bring these perspectives to bear on the substantive issue of control in health and illness.

If a text is defined as any form of meaningful symbolic system, linguistic or otherwise, then *intertextuality* is the process whereby one text engages with other texts (Barthes 1977). For example, there is an intertextual relation between Shakespeare's *Hamlet* and the Tom Stoppard play *Rosenkrantz and Guildenstern are Dead*. As we watch the latter, we make reference to the former, and see allusions and new perspectives, while we also recognize the ironicization of Shakespeare's themes of reason and madness in the intertextual context of the late twentieth century. In a non-linguistic medium, the text which is constituted from the traffic light sequences at road junctions (which depend upon our understanding the meaning of different colours) plays against other texts, from the *Highway Code* to movies involving chase sequences. This play of text on text is endless; there can always be other points of reference for a text. At the simplest level, a dictionary definition refers to other textual elements (words), which in turn are defined by other elements. Similarly, this book makes reference to other texts, which in turn make other references, *ad infinitum*. The development of hypertextual and hypermedia software provides the technology for infinite intertextuality, in which not only books but films, music and other texts play in a limitless web, connected via a click on a hypertextual link (Landow 1992). Three propositions develop the relevance for social analysis of this notion of intertextuality.

1. In the study of the social, the primary unit of analysis is the *text*, which may be writing, bodily or social practice, or subjective sense-of-self, to which meaning may be ascribed. Texts are the product of human activity; as such they are created within the flow of history, yet they are fragmentary, they are continually reread and have no single or final meaning.

2. Texts engage with each other productively, and in this *intertextuality*, meaning comes into being, is sustained, distorted, obscured or reintroduced. In isolation, a text has no meaning, it is only in relation to other texts (including the text which is the reader) that meaning arises. Concomitantly, the capacity for humans to engage *meaningfully* with the social world – that is, to understand and to contribute to that world – is intertextual, a function of a subjectivity which is itself textual and not prior to textuality. Subjectivity is a consequence of the accretion of texts, including texts constituted from reflection (thoughts, desires, memories), which play together to define and delimit a sense of sense. I will return to this in much greater depth in the second part of this book.

3. The 'meaning' of a text is not intrinsic. It can be understood as constructed where texts collide, or more specifically, in a text's *frame*, that is, at the boundary of that which distinguishes and bounds it from what it is not. In Derrida's *The Truth in Painting* (1987b), he demonstrates that power – in the sense of authority and the right to speak 'the truth' – is a consequence of a text's *frame*: to write the limits of a text is a political act. But framing a text is always provisional, subject to challenge and renegotiation, and is always in the process of being achieved.

This notion of a frame is rather different from that developed in Goffman's (1974) *Frame Analysis*, in which a frame is to be understood as the sense-making definitions of situations, by which an individual comes to organize her experience (1974: 10–13). In Goffman's perspective, frames are phenomenological and not concerned with social organization or with social inequity (ibid.: 13–14). Derrida's (1987b) analysis of the 'frame' of a text as the place at which power acts is necessarily social, bearing upon issues of control and resistance. Further, it is more than just the sense-making work of an individual, it can *be* that 'individual' inasmuch as it is at the frame of a text that subjectivity is fabricated.

There are a number of further implications which follow from these propositions, which are worth exploring before turning to look at some instances in health care which will be subjected to this analysis. First, in intertextual approaches, the emphasis is upon the reader rather than the writer: a displacement of great significance for understanding power, knowledge and resistance. While texts are written by humans, their writers' *authorship* is provisional: authority is observable only at its site of action; that is, at the site of reading. Another way of putting this is to say that authority (the capacity to be acknowledged as 'speaking the truth') can never be possessed absolutely, it is always *achieved* and subject to resistance and challenge. The meaning of a text is always provisional, contingent upon how and by whom it is read.

Second, intertextuality contributes endlessly not only to knowledge or 'ideology', but also to that special text which we call 'subjectivity' or sense-of-self. Using the notion of *framing* to explore this further, subjectivity comes to be seen as something dynamic, always in flux as intertextual readings contribute to a continuous process of *becoming-a-self.* Deleuze and Guattari (1984, 1988) describe this in their notion of a 'nomadic subjectivity' potentially free to wander through textuality, although always drawn to one framing (plateau) or another. In the data which will be examined in a moment, on hospital discharge decisions, this is precisely what is happening, as the protagonists are framed as 'subjects' in one way or another.

But third, this is not to imply that an intertextual subjectivity is free to become whatever it may. In practice, framings are constrained in all sorts of ways. For Lyotard (1988), oppositional politics can be understood as a play of texts, what he calls 'phrases in dispute', all seeking to gain authority over the others. When one phrase gains ascendancy, it is by the *denial* of the intertextuality which might enable opposing discourses to 'prove' their own positions. As such, it becomes what Lyotard named the *'differend'*, a marker of the violence which is done in the name of discourse, the 'victimization' of other texts (1988: 9). A differend works by divesting others of the capacity to speak authoritatively or authentically; it is thus the constraining of intertextuality. Such constraint on intertextuality is necessarily imposed from outside of the discourse itself – by the threat of sanctions or through the use of other resources in the psychological or social world of the subject. Medical dominance, patriarchy, religious fundamentalism are all examples of *differends* – authentications of 'reality' which appear based on 'truth' because they deny alternative readings, and ultimately dependent upon the violence of technologies of power.

This position is congruent with Derrida's (1976) notion of *logocentrism*, the privileging of one version of the world such that it becomes possible for a speaker to be accredited with the capacity to speak the 'truth' (*logos*). Once a *logos* is established, then other versions or interpretations become far harder to articulate, because their claims to truth are now brought into question. Readers will note that Lyotard's analysis in terms of *differends* emphasizes *coercive* power. This is somewhat different from Foucault's analysis, which considers disciplinary rather than coercive power to be typical of the modern period (Foucault 1980b: 116–19). For Lyotard, while power may be mediated by knowledge, the right to claim 'knowledge' derives from the possession of power, and when the foundation of such knowledge is openly challenged, those in authority may exercise a more naked power, one which victimizes and silences its opponent. Lyotard's version of power is much more negative than the 'creative' power of Foucault. In this book, coercive and the disciplinary aspects of power will both be acknowledged, and this will be explored in the case studies which form the latter part of this chapter.

In summary, the creation of a *differend* is an act of power which works at the margin or limit of a text. It frames that text (which may be a book or a social practice or a subjectivity), fabricating distance between author and object, self and other, what is and what is not. Deconstruction identifies these framings, exploring the achievement of *differends*. As a strategy, it upsets the accepted definitions, and looks not only at the content of a text (which is created only in relation to its framing), but through the positioning of the limits of text, how it is framed in relationship to that which is beyond. What is excluded is thus as important as what is included in a text or textual practice. Deconstruction reintroduces what has been left outside the frame.

To illustrate these theoretical propositions, I shall take an example from my observation of surgical ward rounds, to explore a contested region: the decision over post-operative discharge.

Framing the Text: Decisions over Discharge from Hospital

Discharge from hospital marks the collision of two realms, that of the medical environment dominated by biomedicine, and a realm in which home, family and 'normal' life provide the primary textualities. The 'stripping' of identity (Goffman 1968) or, perhaps more accurately, the fabrication of an alternate identity as patient (de Swaan 1990) at the outset of a bout of hospitalization has been noted in the literature, but less attention has been paid to discharge from hospital. Decisions over discharge are considered in the medical literature to be primarily technical. However, just as other aspects of engagement between patients and health professionals are social activities (Fox 1993a, 1993b, Nettleton 1992, Roberts 1985, Silverman 1983), discharge from hospital takes place within a social context, and judgements by all involved concerning discharge will never be free of 'social' components. As such, these judgements are tied up with the power and authority of those who make them, and decisions over discharge may be one way in which doctors sustain their control over interactions with patients.

Discharge from hospitalization is not, in law, a medical decision. Any patient, if fit enough, may choose to discharge her/himself at any time, 'against medical advice'. However, from the way in which discharge decisions are made, one might be led to believe that doctors are autocrats with absolute control over whether a patient stays in hospital or leaves. How is it that doctors can sustain this impression? Simplistically, one might argue that patients consign their autonomy to those who have responsibility for their care, acknowledging that specialist knowledge is sufficient warrant for this infringement of self-determination. But this assumes a consensual model of medical authority, which social scientists have challenged; medical interactions are seen as conflictual, based on a variety of perspectives which vie for dominance. So *how* do doctors persuade patients to accept their version of reality over others?

This issue is of particular relevance following elective surgery. Consider the different phases of hospitalization for such procedures. Before surgery, patients have chosen to come into hospital, and placed themselves under the authority of their surgeon. After the procedure has been carried out, and if the surgery is designated a 'success' by surgeon and other staff, the surgeon's version of reality is substantiated by the claims that the patient is 'cured' or ameliorated, in turn sustaining her or his authority to make such definitions. Yet the patient is often now demonstrably 'ill': the effects of surgery and anaesthesia having led elective patients to be considerably less well than upon admission (Fox 1994). This iatrogenic illness is acceptable up to a point, but the surgeon's authority is now open to challenge, because it is as a consequence of her or his actions that the patient remains in hospital. The claims of the 'success' of the surgery are jeopardized by the continuing presence of the post-operative patient on the ward.

As time passes following surgery, the patient's condition usually improves and a surgeon is faced with a conflict, between discharging another 'success', and ensuring a patient is sufficiently recovered to be safely released from her or his gaze. The patient may seize on this conflict, to reassert her or his rights, to quit the uncomfortable environment of the hospital for home, family and 'normality'. The period leading up to discharge may thus be a time of difficult decisions, and of negotiation between doctor and patient, as the latter begin to redefine their situation within texts which are non-medical and relate to their biographical continuity. Surgeons face the possibility in such a situation that the definition of the situation will be inscribed in non-medical textualities, thereby losing control of the decision, and potentially of their authority over it.

To examine the ways in which doctors negotiate this difficult time, I shall consider some data from an ethnographic study of surgery undertaken by the author (Fox 1992). A number of post-operative ward rounds were observed on a general surgical ward and a gynaecology ward at two large teaching hospitals in the UK, and some of the interactions explicitly concerned discharge following surgery. The following analysis will not seek to achieve external validity or 'generalizability' (Lincoln and Guba 1985) through reports of a wide variety of encounters (from a post-structuralist position such claims of validity are merely rhetorical). Rather, three engagements where there is potential contestation of the decision to discharge will be explored using the perspective developed earlier. Each is relatively brief, but even so, they contain great richness in terms of the readings which the participants bring to the engagement.

Extract A: 'Fit or not fit?'

The first interaction occurred between surgeon Mr D and patient Mr Y during a post-operative ward round. The surgeon has a difficult decision to make, exemplifying the conflict of definitions of the patient as healed and yet iatrogenically 'ill'.

> *(Mr D, the junior staff and the researcher gather round Mr Y's bed)*
> *Mr D: (to patient, looking at chart)* Hallo Mr Y. Well we want to send you home, but I don't like that raised temperature.
> *Patient Y:* No.
> *Mr D:* I don't know what can be causing it. We've cultured the wound and there's no infection there. I just don't know what's causing it ... Are things ready for you to go home?
> *Patient Y:* Yes, my wife can come and collect me today.
> *Mr D:* Can you go to bed, and she can look after you?
> *Patient Y:* Yes.
> *Mr D:* I don't like that raised temperature. Phone your wife and you can go home now.
> *Patient Y:* Thank you very much.

It is worth beginning this first deconstruction by thinking about the textualities involved. The number of texts which might be discerned in this engagement is potentially endless (because of course, as readers we ourselves engage intertextually and thus productively with this text (Fox 1995c), and there can be no 'final' or ultimately correct reading). But amongst others, we may identify:

(a) The body of the patient, and the operation on Mr Y
(b) The context of the surgical ward
(c) Surgery as a discipline/skill/profession
(d) Mr D's professional occupation
(e) Mr Y's history as a patient, including the chart held by Mr D
(f) Mr Y's biography, and his home and life outside the hospital

Some of these are literally texts, while others are 'social' or 'body' texts, and the impact of each will depend on its framing. However, the deconstruction is not wholly unwieldy. What are of interest are those frames which mediate the power relations of the encounter, in other words, those which serve as *differends*, violently disrupting the free flow of intertextuality, and working as a text's frame, at the delimitation of a text or where two or more texts collide.

What might be the *differends* here: the framings which write Mr Y and Mr D, silencing other voices, other textualities? There is the ward, and there is the bed which Mr Y is sitting upon while Mr D and the rest of us stand over him. There is biomedicine, with its definitions and mystique of language. But perhaps the framing which is of greatest rhetorical use here is Mr Y's chart, on which is inscribed a text of his body in terms of temperature, heart rate etc. The chart has a very literal frame, in that it covers the period of Mr Y's hospitalization; beyond this temporal frame past and future cease to have any relevance. And it has a second metaphorical frame in its concerns with biomedically defined vital signs.

Mr D holds the chart, he is in control of it and Mr Y does not get to see it. Mr D uses the chart's frame to frame the opening remarks, to mark out his authority over Mr Y's disposal. The chart frames Mr Y in terms of time and the signs recorded there. Nothing outside the frame of the chart is to be considered now, and the chart's biomedical framing sets the parameters within which the decision is to be. Anything which is beyond the chart is excluded; Mr Y is written by the chart, he is the chart.

While this *differend* supplies Mr D's control of the situation, this framing is provisional and Mr D admits this himself, because the chart reveals something disturbing about Mr Y: he has a raised temperature, a possible complication which will need to be resolved before discharge. Mr D *doesn't like* this raised temperature. Why? Firstly, because it means Mr Y *is not fit*, not fit for discharge. Secondly, (and he uses the identical phrase a second time), Mr D doesn't like it because it means Mr Y *does not fit* the framing which he wants to impose, of Mr Y as healed, an ex-patient, ready for discharge.

But Mr D wants this annoying temperature not to fit, to be excluded from his decision-making. So he must victimize it, creating a new *differend* to exclude it. Raised temperatures are things patients have, but Mr Y (Mr D wishes to demonstrate) is a non-patient, a success of surgery, he should have none of the attributes of a patient. To construct the *differend*, Mr D tests the limits of the text which is Mr Y and his raised temperature: the temperature is nothing to do with the operation ('there's no infection'), it is irrelevant ('I just don't know what's causing it'), Mr Y is ready to go home, his wife is ready to take him away, he will continue his recuperation at home, he is physically capable of action ('phone your wife'). Mr D disallows the raised temperature any rights to define Mr Y. Mr Y is written as an ex-patient; no doubt in time, he will be written up.

Extract B: 'Stitched up'

In the second extract, discharge of patient S is to be postponed, for a dramatic reason. Following an abdominal procedure, Mrs S's wound had burst. For surgeon Mr O, a 'success' of surgery, due to have been discharged, has been unexpectedly transformed into a 'complication', which is all too visible. For Mrs S, the expectation is now a longer stay in hospital.

Patient S is sitting in an armchair, and looks very unhappy
Surgeon Mr O: Hallo, Mrs S, well we were going to send you home yesterday weren't we, and thank the God Almighty we didn't.
Patient S: (quietly) No.
Mr O: Well, we just don't know why this happened; there's no infection, no haematoma, nothing at all to cause this. You were up and walking ...?
Nurse: Yes she was walking about, and went to the lavatory and was straining, and then ...
Mr O: ... Yes, I hear there was small intestine hanging out. Well, you've had a nasty time, and we'll keep you in for ten days.
Patient S: (aghast) Ten ... days ...?
Mr O: Yes, but there's absolutely nothing the matter inside, we don't know why this happened, so we'll keep you in for ten days.

Mr O had probably never expected to see patient S as an in-patient again. She was out of the frame which she has occupied as a hospital patient, excluded and written down as a success of surgery. Now she is back again, and Mr O is faced with a difficult explanation, of why this success has so dramatically returned to haunt him. How could he have made what was effectively an incorrect decision to discharge this patient, whose very presence indicates she was insufficiently recovered to be sent home? Is he to blame for a framing which could potentially have had disastrous consequences had the wound burst once Mrs S had left hospital?

Mrs S's sutures supply Mr O with his *differend*, a new frame of reference which denies alternative readings and sustains his authority. What was inside has come out, it has burst through the stitches he put in place to frame Mrs S's success, and yet 'there's absolutely nothing the matter inside'. Mr O cannot be held responsible: nothing he did – allowing infection or a blood vessel to leak – can be found to explain the burst sutures. Mrs S was showing all the signs of recovery, walking about the ward, using the lavatory. Now Mrs S has been stitched up again, what should be inside is back in place, and the wound sutures frame her surgery once again as a success – albeit of one who has suffered complications.

In such circumstances, Mr O has little difficulty renegotiating a new discharge date, a very conservative distance ahead, so no new circumstance can challenge his authority to dispose of his patient appropriately. Mrs S is very much the victim of this *differend*, which denies any role for Mr O in this episode. Mrs S's exertions had caused her stitches to burst – now she must suffer the consequences. All that matters is that what is framed by the stitches remains so; Mrs S's biography is of no concern.

Extract C: 'I'll ask the questions'

Lyotard's analysis (1988) of the creation of *differends* emphasizes the unequal nature of these power plays, dependent on all sorts of imbalances in resources between actors. Whereas patient Y was compliant (perhaps because he was getting his desired discharge), and patient S is literally and metaphorically stitched up, in the following extract, surgeon Mrs A has to work hard to sustain her authority against challenge, and it could be argued that she is left with little resource other than her role as the decision-maker. Mrs A had previously implied that patient Z, an old lady whose recovery had been slower than expected after a major gynaecological procedure, might be discharged on the day this encounter took place.

Surgeon Mrs A: Hallo, Mrs Z, I think you can go home on Monday.
Patient Z: On Monday, not today?

> *Mrs A:* No, I think we'll keep you in till Monday. *(to house officer)* Doctor, can you listen to her tummy ... *(to patient)* Where do you live Mrs Z?
> *Patient Z:* In (...)
> *Mrs A:* On your own?
> *Patient Z:* Yes, but I've arranged for my sisters to come over to me ...
> *Mrs A:* ...Yes. *(to house officer)* Does that sound OK?
> *House Officer:* Yes, it's OK.
> *Patient Z:* They're nurses. They're not actually working any more, but they're qualified nurses ...
> *Mrs A:* Yes, you can go on Monday. *(turns away and walks off)*

Patient Z immediately challenges surgeon Mrs A's opening gambit, because it is at variance with a previous expectation. In response, Mrs A initiates a two-pronged interrogation. She asks the house officer to gather data for her to use within a textuality concerning recovery. He is told to listen to Mrs Z's abdominal sounds, and is then asked to confirm whether they are normal. However the significance of this information is not passed back to patient Z or discussed with the house officer. Simultaneously, the surgeon begins a search procedure concerning Mrs Z's situation as a potential ex-patient: where she lives; if she has carers. Mrs Z seizes on this to try to establish her own *differend* concerning the care she will receive at home, challenging Mrs A's assessment that she needs hospital care.

Mrs A is apparently left with few resources to sustain her authority. Neither line of questioning has provided data which supports the deferral of discharge. Even her question and answer strategy has been subverted by the patient's information about her carers. Yet she may resort to her status: she is the one standing up, who can walk away, leaving Mrs Z in bed; she is the one asking the questions and making the decisions. Mrs A ends by baldly restating her first utterance, and now it can be seen that her initial statement was intended to seize the initiative, to assert from the start her framing of herself as the decision-maker, and the patient as the fortunate recipient of this benign authority. In this situation, power validates itself, its victim remains a victim.

Frames, Health and Control

It is clear from these three ethnographic extracts that conflict can arise when patients negotiate with their surgeons over discharge from hospital. It is of relevance that this conflict is to be found at the demarcation of a role change from patient to person, in other words at the point of the *framing* of patienthood. Becoming a patient entails both a change of subjectivity (from person to patient), and entry into a status in which that subjectivity is influenced by medical authority. Leaving that status may mean escaping from medical authority, but that does not mean that authority is relinquished without a struggle.

This account introduces power into the equation in a way which is absent from other accounts of the patient role, including the consensual functionalism of Parsons (1951), in which 'society' somehow oversees the rights and responsibilities accorded to patents, or the dramaturgical model of Goffman in which institutionalization entails a 'stripping of identity' or 'loss of self' (Goffman 1968: 28–32) to aid patient management. Discharge from hospital is not simply a matter of physical displacement. Nor is it always merely the re-establishment of subjectivity in some reflexive process of 'getting back to normal life'.

The analysis which has been undertaken here suggests that the social processes involved in discharge are as much tied up with medical authority and power as any which take place between patients and health professionals. Surgeons use their authority to frame the subjectivity of their patients up to the moment of discharge, and where necessary do this through manipulations of texts which have been considered here as *differends*. We might conclude that medical authority owes part of its puissance to the framing acts of patienthood.

There is a well-established corpus of work to suggest this is true for the entry into the status of patient (Kleinman 1980, Tuckett *et al.* 1985); this case material suggests the same is true for departure from that state. To explore this proposition further, I want to take a look at a range of other empirical materials bearing upon the framing of health/illness encounters. These derive from the anthropological study of health and are associated with a perspective quite different from that developed here: the theory of the *rite de passage*.

It has been argued by a number of prominent anthropologists including Victor Turner and Mary Douglas, that rites of passage are present in many cultures, and are particularly associated with changes in status. First developed by Van Gennep in 1909, the concept of the *rite de passage* ascribes a tri-partite character to rituals of this kind: a phase of separation which signifies detachment of a person from her or his current social grouping or status, a 'liminal' phase in which the subject's status is ambiguous, and is often associated with licence or unusual behaviour, and finally a reintegrative phase in which the subject becomes part of a new group or is ascribed a new status (Turner 1968: 94–5). The order of phases is crucial for the ritual to be seen as successful: get some detail wrong and the whole process needs to start over. The passage through the ritual over a period of time is often accompanied by movements in space, to confirm the correct proceeding of the rite.

In the West, *rites de passage* have been identified in a range of ceremonials, particularly associated with the life course (christening, circumcision, *bar-mitzvah*, funerals) and with changes in status such as weddings or coronations (Bocock 1974: 118ff.). Helman has described hospitalization as a rite of passage possessing a phase of separation (Goffman's 'stripping'), a transition and then a reincorporation (Helman 1984: 132). Some caution is needed however: while such a description could be associated with many activities, it is unclear whether this amounts to saying much more than that most things have a beginning, a middle and an end (Gluckman 1962: 9).

Anthropologists have focused much attention on the liminal phase, when subjects are betwixt and between. Some anthropologists have recognized the rights which liminal subjects possess (for example, in the carnivalesque inversion of normal behaviour), while Douglas notes that subjects in liminal states are often seen as dangerous and polluting because they do not fit into accepted social categories (Douglas 1966: 96). I want to suggest that a focus on this phase is the wrong emphasis: what are more interesting are the phases of separation and reintegration, because here we see at work the authority of those who control the ritual. It is only because those who set the rites in progress have the capacity to claim the truth about what the ritual signifies, that they can have any force. A number of non-western examples of health-related rites may be cited to explore this argument further.

The rite of *liengu* among the Bakweri of the Cameroons (Ardener 1972) was enacted to cure a seizure which characteristically affects a woman causing her to faint over the fireplace, knocking out one of the stones supporting the cooking pot (an occurrence shocking because of its subversion of the normal role of the woman as cook and housekeeper). The *liengu* doctor (usually male) kills a black cock and sprinkles its blood in the hole left by the displaced hearthstone. The woman is then secluded in a hut, taught the secret *liengu* language and given a new *liengu* name. After several months she is taken and submerged in a deep stream, where she becomes a familiar of the water-spirits which caused the seizure. Subsequently she is immune from further attack from these spirits. Ardener suggested that while from a male perspective this is a medical rite, from the women's viewpoint *liengu* is a resolution of the contradiction of living both in a culture (defined by men) and in nature (the water-spirit world). *Liengu* rites are at once both medical and concerned with resolving the contradictions faced by girls about to enter marriage: between their perceived 'wild' nature and their subordination by men (Ardener 1972: 153).

Turner witnessed many rites associated with healing among the Ndembu. *Nkula*, a rite concerned to make a barren woman fertile, he noted was etymologically related to the word for 'to mature', a word also attached to women's various passages through menarche, first pregnancy, multiparity and menopause. The felling of a tree and the sacrifice of a cock, Turner suggested, symbolize the cutting away of the masculinity of the barren woman, returning her to the role of normal wife (Turner 1968: 86–7). The rite of *Ihamba*, concerned with the casting out of an affliction caused by a displeased ancestor, displays the feature common to other rites, that the subject, having passed through the rite, becomes an adept, and may himself become a practitioner of the healing (ibid.: 197). Within his structural-functionalist paradigm, Turner concluded that 'the typical development of a ritual sequence is from the public expression of a wish to cure a patient and redress breaches in the social structure, through exposure of hidden animosities, to the renewal of social bonds' (Ibid.: 272). He argued that as with other rites of passage among Ndembu, rites of healing resolved the specific tensions in that society resulting from the contradiction of matriliny (property descent through the female line) and virilocality (the settling of a new married couple in the man's village), as well as other pressures from modernization (ibid.: 273).

Having explored the concepts of the frame and the *differend* earlier in this chapter, a different understanding of these various rites may be suggested. What seems important is the emphasis on rites which will put right what is seen as a dangerous breach of cultural norms (a failure to carry out normal social duties, barrenness, challenge to male authority). In each case, the subject submits to the authority of the rite-master, who will proclaim – after the ritual is complete – that the problem has been resolved and the subject is reintegrated. The meaning of the rite lies not in the liminal state (indeed, the behaviour or arrangements during this phase are often bizarre), but in the imposition of a separation and then the proclamation of reintegration. The ritual works because the aberrant element is subdued by the authority of the culture as personified by the person or people leading the rite. It is a demonstration of power and control, which silences opposition to the norms or values of the social group. The liminal phase is of significance only in its intervention between the two key phases of separation and reintegration at which points the cultural authority is exerted.

These examples from non-western settings portray features both of the power of the frame (the start and finish of the ritual intervention) and the *differend* which silences the resistance to cultural authority. These rites are indeed acts of violence which demonstrate the blatant exercise of coercive power. That they may appear collaborative (the subjects being active and willing participants in the ritual) does not diminish the extent to which they are victims (to use Lyotard's phrase), whose acts of resistance are crushed by the weight of tradition. Turning back to the case study of discharge from hospital, we see elements of this despotism in the actions of the surgeons, who silence opposition and bring to bear the full power of medical authority to ensure the move from patient to person is under their control.

The Force of the Differend

Using the Derridean analysis of frames illustrates two elements of the argument which I am developing. The first concerns conflict, the second, consensus.

Concerning conflict, in the study of the meanings surrounding the discharge of surgical patients, conflicting texts on the subjectivity of the patient (deriving from medical and biographical frames) come into play. In deconstruction, the 'inequality' between such texts becomes clearer, and we can begin to understand why some texts become dominant at the expense of others. Firstly, the framing of texts which enables them to 'make sense' takes place in a context: the impinging universe of potential textualities, including the hospital's architecture and routines; the institution of biomedicine; the disciplines of medicine and nursing; and the biographical and medical history of the patient. Secondly, while new texts may be introduced to support one or another reading, the ability to introduce such texts depends on an environment which is supportive to 'other voices', and often, such an environment does not exist. Framing of texts sometimes leads to the creation of victims: those who are unable to speak in the face of a *differend,* a textual framing which violently refuses to permit alternative readings.

Concerning discharge, we have seen this violence in action. Medical authority is the capacity to choose the framing of a patient's subjectivity, to include and exclude those texts which suit or do not, to serve the *differend* by which the patient is to be discharged or is to remain a patient a little longer. Participants in these exchanges, buoyed by claims to authenticity, draw upon resources: the discipline of biomedicine and the rights to self-determination of the human subject amongst others. When interpretations of events cease to be consensual, the achievement of outcomes depends on a naked exercising of power in the creation of *differ-ends.* Looking at some of the 'health'-related rituals from other cultures demonstrates the assertion of power, particularly in the separation of ritual subjects from the rest of their society, and then their reintegration at a time and place which is determined by tradition rather than the subjects' own volition.

However, we must not overemphasize the conflict and the victimization at the expense of a recognition of the importance of consensus. The surgeons in the case study were not acting maliciously, but in the best interest of their patients, at least as they saw the matter. Their decisions were grounded in their experience and based – at least in part – upon evidence. If the three extracts selected here demonstrated the action of *differends*, then others would suggest a much greater consensus between surgeon and patient (albeit, usually when the surgeon is supporting a decision to discharge the patient that day!). This is important, because much of the time, we go along with the framings which are imposed, the 'truth' or *logos* which interprets the world in a particular way. I do not question the notions of the movement of the sun across the sky as I look out of my window at the afternoon turning to evening, nor do I necessarily see the cityscape as a blot on a natural landscape. The children in the art exhibition had accepted the ministrations of their teachers who showed them how to imitate impressionism or post-impressionist artists.

Foucault has pointed to the productive character of power, which can feel good, safe or liberating. As we learn our history or sociology or biology we are initiated into a shared culture (Foucault 1988a: 162). Furthermore, it is constitutive of a sense-of-self, of who we are and what it is to be human (Foucault 1988b: 49). Framing the world, even though it is an act of power as Derrida points out, comes to *feel* like a Goffmanesque framing in which meaning and sense become possible. In short, framing may be something which is perceived not as a malignant process of imposition, but as a benign liberation into a world which makes sense. This of course, was at the root of traditional models of education (from the Latin *educare*: to 'lead out'), which were seen as civilizing the raw and anarchic material of the child.

This, I want to suggest, is why the body, health and illness seem so much like givens. Anatomy, physiology and the human sciences have fabricated ways of thinking (frames) about these entities which are 'good to think'; they provide ways of thinking about these important aspects of life which are both culturally satisfying and operationally useful. The success of biomedicine is not just based upon acts of power (disciplinary or coercive) but upon its operational success in predicting important things like recovery from illness, ageing or death. So efforts to challenge and resist these bodies of knowledge are likely to be hard to achieve.

One way forward is through the kind of deconstructive work which has been undertaken in this chapter, focusing on the interstices, the points where the frames become obvious, where *differends* silence alternative voices. As a strategy, deconstruction is thus not only a methodology of qualitative data analysis, but also a political tool which opposes authoritarian exercises of power in the denial of intertextuality. As such, the deconstruction of discharge decisions has clear political implications for patients and health-care professionals around interactions over discharge, and at other points where subjectivities as patients and professionals are fabricated. The emphasis on violence and victimization paints a less rosy picture of the way power works than those in traditional analyses of such 'negotiations'. More generally, it suggests a way of exposing the silencing of alternatives. Once exposed, *differends* lose their power to silence; like petty dictators they are shown up as bullies and charlatans.

Deconstruction opens up the frame, questioning why some things are included and others excluded. Of course, at the same time, it creates its own framings, and any deconstruction can be subjected to similar interrogation itself. As such, deconstructive work is never final or complete: there is always another possible reading. Were this not the case, it would itself be a *differend*, violently refusing other voices. With this in mind, the strategy can supply the possibility of resistance, for new framings: of subjectivities which can 'become other', of voices which until now had been silent.

From an intertextual perspective, there are an infinite number of texts which may be written and read as we live out the social world. The undifferentiated events which make up the flow of history provide the raw material for this endless play of intertextuality. At the same time, 'history' (the texts we call the past and the present) is the product of intertextuality. Events, bodies and selves are written and read, as they are framed to provide meaningful textualities. Yet the number of texts which comprise the shared social world are often quite limited; there is not the massive proliferation of meaning which intertextuality implies. To move *beyond health* may mean removing those limits, seeking out new plays of text on text, new ways of thinking. In the next two chapters, further deconstruction explores the frames which have been established around health and care.

2
Space, Time and Health

The tension between 'agency' and 'structure' has dogged sociology for much of its history. Indeed this dualism may be at the heart of what makes sociology a discipline in its own right, separated from social psychology on one hand, and economics and politics on the other. Within the discipline, some theorists emphasized structure, others agency. Grand schemes have been proposed to resolve this tension, from Giddens' theory of structuration (1984) in which agency is seen as constitutive of structure, while structure is the medium and context of agency, to Foucauldian approaches (which I consider in chapter 4), which have claimed to demonstrate agentic practices as the source of power and social order (Silverman 1985, Eckermann 1997: 155).

Post-structuralism has, as its name implies, largely rejected notions of social structure as determining, or as anything other than an epiphenomenon of systems of thought and the associated regimes of power and control. In this chapter, I shall employ a post-structuralist or postmodern take on power and control, to demonstrate what this kind of perspective entails, and to set the scene for the second part of this book. As will become clear, the approach I am developing acknowledges that power and control may operate through systems of thought and knowledge about the world and the body, but that these systems can be subverted. As such it will suggest – paradoxically – both the flimsiness of these constructions (that 'structure' is not really structural in any meaningful sense of the word), and that mechanisms of power may be unsubtle, and often (as in the examples offered in the previous chapter) dependent upon crude acts of coercion: threatening or even imposing acts of violence on their subjects.

This chapter will consider two features of existence (generally, and specifically concerning health and illness) which at first sight may not seem 'social' at all: space and time. I am going to show how these two constructs – independently of whether or not they are attributes of the physical universe – are vectors of power and control in the realm of the social, yet are also media in which resistance is possible. The capacity of these two elements – space and time – to affect us will be seen to be based in ways of thinking about the world. Thinking space and time in other ways can open up new possibilities for action.

As such, the analysis in this chapter will demonstrate the central theme of this book: the potentiality in all of us to be freed from the constraints of embodiment, and move *beyond health*. In the following sections on space and time, I shall use data from a number of sources, including my research on surgery and older adults' experiences of care.

Space: Health and the Built Environment

Hospitals are the modern cathedrals of health and illness. Just as Christian cathedrals have architectural as well as spiritual significance, and just as these aspects are intimately associated, so it is with the hospital. The impact of the spaces of the built environment upon health and health care have been documented by many authors, and a number of the approaches are discernible in these studies.

First, there have been studies of the impact of health-care environment upon perceptions, experiences and well-being, including patients' recovery. For example, ward design has been analysed in terms of the creation of a 'healing' (Biley 1993) or 'therapeutic' (Cotton and Geraty 1984) environment, or in terms of staff preferences (Trites *et al.* 1970). For such writers, space is important as a background or context against which social and psychological processes occur.

Interactionist studies, second, have examined the more direct impact of architecture on the engagements between people who inhabit the spaces. Rawlings (1989) found problems of communication between personnel working in a surgical sterilization unit due to physical boundaries in layout, while the spatial allocation of patients in a casualty department was analysed in terms of doctor/nurse interactions by Hughes (1988).

Third, structuralist approaches in anthropology and sociology examined how spaces and movements within spaces mirror or otherwise symbolically represent the activities which go on in them. Turner's (1968) study of the Ndembu people explored *rites de passage* associated with sickness which entailed complex movements, while Ardener considered the use of spatial isolation in the *liengu* rite (described in more detail in the previous chapter) used to heal seizures among the Cameroonian Bakweri

(Ardener 1972). Rosengren and DeVault (1963) examined the spatial arrangements of obstetrics, while passing mention of the spaces of surgery is made in Hirschauer's (1991) analysis of surgical bodies. Studies within this tradition may distinguish between 'ritual' and instrumental activities, and seek to disclose a 'deep structure' beneath the surface manifestations of the interactions (Levi-Strauss 1986).

Cutting across these interactionist and structuralist explanations, Goffman's approach acknowledged the symbolic or dramaturgical use of space when he contrasted front (public) and back (private or exclusive) space (Goffman 1959). Back spaces are those exclusively occupied by staff or 'insiders' (doctors and nurses in a hospital, actors and stage crew in a theatre, priest and acolytes at a church service) and the normal rules of behaviour or decorum of an institution which invites the 'public' into its front spaces may be absent or moderated in the back space. Back spaces are necessarily defined in opposition to front spaces, and are both exclusionary (of outsiders) and inclusive in that they define 'insiders' and facilitate different kinds of interactions to go on within them. Definitions of spaces as 'front' and 'back' are contingent and mutable, usually at the discretion of the 'insiders'.

While Goffman's model focuses on power and its mediation through features such as the built environment, it is deterministic: denying possibilities of resistance or redefinition (particularly in the context of the 'total institution' (Goffman 1968)). The post-structuralist or postmodern position eschews any notion that the built environment is *determining* of behaviour, or that there is a one-to-one congruity between architecture and the intended function of a space. Post-structuralism is interested in power and its relationship to knowledge, and the built environment may contribute to a 'knowledge' of such things as how to behave, who may behave in certain ways and who is ascribed particular privilege. Such an approach emphasizes the 'reading' of spaces by actors rather than the 'writing' of behavioural imperatives within the physical structure of the built environment. Thus, in certain circumstances, architecture may make available to actors a skein of signs with which they can support their discursive activities. For example, Prior writes that the design of health-care spaces

> ... can be best understood in relation to the discursive practices which are disclosed in their interiors. The architecture of the hospital is therefore inextricably bound up with the forms of medical theorizing and medical practice which were operant [sic] at the hour of their construction ... all subsequent modifications to hospital design can be seen as a product of alterations in medical discourse. (Prior 1988: 110)

Spaces may offer *cues* to actors as to how they might engage with the environment and with others. On the other hand, they are not themselves 'discursive', in that they may be read in ways other than those in which they had been 'written'. The built environment is adaptable, and in no way *determines* action or behaviour. To understand the significance of space in health and health care we cannot depend upon analysis of the spaces themselves, but must look at the meanings ascribed to the spaces, and how the spaces are used to facilitate behaviours and routines.

The surgical operating theatre or operating room (henceforth OR) is one of the most inaccessible 'backspaces' (to apply Goffman's terminology) of the modern hospital, often signposted in code to further reduce the possibility of a casual and unwelcome visitor. The fabrication of spaces which help to exclude outsiders may thus not only separate the OR physically from an otherwise relatively public space – the hospital – but permit interactions within the back space of the OR to be distinct from those which go on elsewhere in the building, freed from the intrusion of (conscious) patients and other outsiders. An exploration of this space yields some fascinating insights into the interaction between physical spaces and social behaviour (Fox 1992). While there is diversity in the layout of ORs, Figure 2.1 may be used as an illustration of a common design with which many are congruent if not identical.

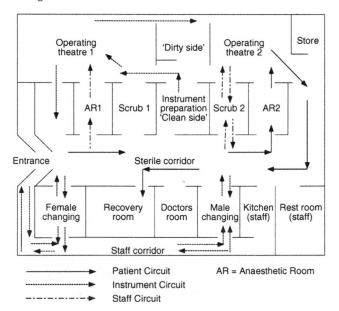

Figure 2.1 Operating Theatre Layout at 'General' Hospital
(N.B. for simplicity, movements are not duplicated for both theatres in this suite)

One approach to documenting the spatiality of the OR is that it is arranged around a central core area of the sterile corridor. The entrance to this corridor is clearly marked as off-limits to patients, visitors, and staff not authorized to enter, and forms the principal barrier and boundary to the OR. Nursing staff and porters accompanying patients to theatre use this route. However, most of the personnel based in the OR use a different means of access. Either between the two sets of doors, or via a discreetly marked staff entrance, access is obtained to a staff corridor, which leads to changing rooms. Changing rooms contain washing and toilet facilities, and stocks of sterile clothing. Suitably garbed, personnel are able to enter the sterile corridor via an internal door from the changing rooms. These are the 'back spaces' of this 'back space'.

Associated with the OR are an anaesthetic room and scrub areas, and also instrument preparation and disposal facilities. This area forms the inner sanctum within the OR, to which access is limited to specific personnel. The 'clean side' instrument preparation area is accessible from the sterile corridor, and here sterile instruments from a Central Sterile Supplies Department (CSSD) in the hospital are unpacked and arranged on sterile trolleys which are subsequently wheeled into theatre via a corridor between the ORs. Used instruments are returned to the 'dirty side', often via a hatchway towards the rear of each OR, to be replaced in the containers in which they arrived and returned in due course to the CSSD. Scrub areas contain washing facilities and stocks of sterile gowns, gloves and masks for use by surgeons and scrub nurses.

The other areas comprise a recovery room for post-operative patients, and areas for use by staff: offices for doctors and the theatre sister, a rest room, and equipment stock rooms. The OR is thus virtually autonomous of the hospital, and in some ORs where all day lists are conducted, arrangements are made to provide snack luncheons for staff, obviating the need to leave the OR between 9 a.m. and late afternoon. Telephones situated in the sterile corridor and in the offices, and the bleep system permit limited contact with the outside world to be maintained, although it can also effectively be kept at a distance by claiming pressure of urgent work to be done in the OR. One informant told me how one of the pleasures of working in surgery was the inaccessibility.

Infection Control Nurse: Danger of infection will be used as the excuse for all the expense (of architectural arrangement), but these precautions are also very effective in keeping unwanted people out of theatre.

However, while this description is accurate, the spatial organization of the OR makes sense only in the context of theories of hygiene. Sterility is a key element in organizing activity within the OR area, and can be analysed as three concentric spaces of increasing hygiene.

1. The general environs of the OR, comprising the areas described earlier, and marked out as off-limits to any except those involved in one way or another in the activities of the OR. In this area, some efforts are made to adopt sterile procedures, for example, avoiding contact with surfaces by street clothing or shoes.

2. The OR itself, which may be entered only by those garbed in surgical clothing comprising 'greens' (linen shirt and trousers or skirt), clogs or boots, a cap or surgical hood, and in theory at least, a surgical mask. Clothing supplies are provided in the changing rooms which may be accessed through entrances to the OR complex avoiding the sterile corridor. While clean, the OR – including the operating table and other equipment – are not sterile.

3. The 'sterile field' surrounding the patient, or more precisely, that part of the patient which will be the focus of the surgical procedure. Anyone approaching this area should wear a surgical gown, sterile rubber gloves and a surgical mask. Furthermore, all personnel in this area must first have undergone the ritual of scrubbing the hands and forearms. The gloved hands must not touch anyone or anything which is not sterile, including mask or cap. Patients are considered to be non-sterile, and will be transformed into 'sterile objects' by draping with towelling from neck to toe. Parts of a patient immediately adjacent to the site of the proposed incision area are washed with a disinfectant such as iodine, after which further sterilized towels are draped so as to leave a small rectangular area of skin exposed. A sterile adhesive plastic material may then be stuck to skin and surrounding towels, so that incisions are made through this membrane and underlying skin, enhancing the sterility of the area immediately adjacent to the wound. Towelling may be augmented by a non-porous paper barrier placed under conventional cloth towelling.

The use of towelling or sterile plastic sheeting to create a barrier extends to drapes for any piece of equipment which is to be above an operation, such as an x-ray machine in orthopaedic surgery, or a microscope for plastic surgery. It is worth noting that while most sterile practices are intended to protect the patient from the surgical environment (including personnel), surgical garb may also be a protection for staff against contamination by patients with blood-borne diseases such as hepatitis and HIV.

Those who work in the spaces of the surgical enterprise must learn the rules of the OR, many of which concern the sterility of the theatre and surrounding areas. Asepsis is a technology for the exclusion of infecting agents which might contaminate the sterile inside of the body during surgery, and the development of the built environment of the OR over the past 100 years reflects the developments in antisepsis and asepsis (Trites *et al.* 1970, Fox 1988). It requires that all objects which come into contact with this sterile field (instruments, clothes and bodies) must be as far as possible germ-free, as should the air and other contents of the environment of the surgical operation. In practice of course, complete asepsis is impossible, and the procedures are nowadays usually complemented by pre-operative injections of antibiotics.

The built environment of the OR is thus crucial for this aseptic technique in two ways. Firstly, it demarcates the sterile area from the general septic environment of the hospital. Thus, within the precincts of the OR, sterile practices must be observed, and adherence to rules of dress and behaviour are required of all who inhabit the spaces. Secondly, the OR environment affects the spatial movements of personnel, patients and instruments which are 'permissible' according to rules of sterility. These are partly built into the architecture of the OR; in this sense, the built environment is potentially a 'guarantor' against inadvertent compromise of aseptic procedures. I have called these rules of movement, the 'circuits of hygiene' (Fox 1992).

In Figure 2.1, arrows indicate the direction in which instruments, staff and patients usually move, and these comprise three interdependent circuits of hygiene. There are no rules in the forms of signs or physical impedimenta to govern which directions are permissible, although of course barriers in the form of architectural construction limit possible movements. Yet there are learnt conventions which lay down how staff, patients and instruments may move; it would be considered extremely unusual (and dangerous) were a patient or an instrument to move in an unconventional direction. For example, while the scrub room may be used as a thoroughfare, it is conventional (partly to avoid disturbing patients awaiting anaesthetic induction) that the anaesthetic room is seen as the domain of anaesthetists and their assistant nurses, and is not used by other staff to access the OR, even when no patient is present.

These circuits of hygiene serve to bring together staff (surgeon and other scrub personnel), patient, and instruments in ways which are safe according to aseptic theory. If one or more circuits are compromised then the interaction breaks the rules of hygiene which this theory requires, and the surgical procedure is no longer safe.

Such an analysis might be understood as an architectural *determination* of behaviour, congruent with the proposition implicit in Foucault's (and Foucauldians') discussions of spaces such as the prison, school and work place. Most notably, Foucault's discussion of the Panopticon in prison and hospital design (Foucault 1979) suggests that the built environment made a regime of surveillance possible, and furthermore, that it rendered resistance to this surveillance impossible.

> In organizing 'cells', 'places' and 'ranks', the disciplines create complex spaces which are at once architectural, functional and hierarchical. It is spaces [sic] that provide fixed positions and permit circulation; they carve out individual segments and establish operational links; they mark places and indicate values; they guarantee the obedience of individuals, but also a better economy of time and gesture. (Foucault 1979: 148)

Yet I would reject this determinism. The imperatives of the circuits of hygiene demonstrate how spatiality mediates systems of thought: spatial organization is both enabling and constraining. First, the architecture does not prevent breaches in convention; that such breaches rarely occur is due to socialization and a shared system of thinking about sterility. Second, spaces serve to confer certain rights upon people; in the context of the OR, to cut other people open and generally act in ways unacceptable elsewhere. Step outside (literally or metaphorically) these boundaries, and what is being done becomes dangerous and therefore not to be permitted.

Perhaps it is better to think about the built environment as offering *cues* to behaviour. Spaces may incorporate features of a system of thought, as Prior (1988) suggests, so that they limit the possible movements which can be enacted within them in line with – in the case of the OR – the theory of asepsis. But there is flexibility, permitted movements are not absolute, rather they are conventional and arbitrary. For instance, were humoral theory to have remained in the ascendant, rather than having been superseded by a germ theory of infection, surgical practices would differ, with less emphasis on sterile practice and more upon ambient conditions such as air quality (Fox 1988). The social relations of the hospital cut across the imperatives of spatiality, as I noted on various occasions during my fieldwork. For instance, the legitimacy of an action within the OR may depend upon its author.

> A trainee paramedic went for a coffee-break during an operation. He returned with cups of coffee for consultant anaesthetist Dr B and the researcher.

Dr B: (*to the researcher*) You had better take yours outside. It is only consultants who are allowed to drink their coffee here. *(Field Notes)*

Conventions can be altered:

Surgeon Mr P: At G (a new private hospital), when commissioned, a red line on the floor demarcated sterile areas in the OR. However, the inclusion of the coffee-room within this boundary prevented surgeons' colleagues dropping by for coffee, thus disrupting a convention of hospital sociability. The red line was quickly repainted to exclude the coffee-room from the sterile area.

Finally, the mystique of the OR can rub off on those who work there. Nurses working in the recovery room, within the environs of the OR, felt contaminated by its spatial and symbolic distance from the rest of the hospital.

Nurse A: They (ward nurses) don't like (people who work) in recovery. You're in-between.
Anaesthetic nurse: You're definitely in-between.

The circuits of hygiene contribute to what Laufman (1990) has suggested is a 'covenant' between staff and patient to provide appropriate asepsis and thus 'safe' surgery. They 'guarantee' that the patient arrives at the moment when surgery begins in a condition which is intended to ensure that the operation does not unintentionally increase the 'illness' of the patient through infection. She or he is disinfected and sterile towels are draped. Instruments are sterilized, and the people who are to wield them undergo routines to ensure that as far as possible they do not introduce infecting agents into the wound. These procedures are time-consuming, yet they are recognized as essential. Corners cannot be cut, and the routines are accepted by all involved as legitimate uses of staff time and resources. The circuits routinize these efforts, they remove responsibility from the surgeon for overseeing the entire proceedings, and assure her or him that all has been done to enable healing to take place safely. When the surgeon approaches the operating table, the rhetoric of the circuits of hygiene assures her or him that all has been done according to the rules of asepsis, and that she or he may operate with maximum certainty that her or his intervention will not endanger the patient by infection. Without this assurance, the intervention would be classed not as surgery, but as physical assault.

The built environment of the OR is thus not *essential* to surgery. One surgeon in the study commented that he could operate in the middle of a cornfield, and it would probably be a lot safer. But the architecture is a reminder to staff to adhere to sterile procedure. It can be 'read', and contributes to the routines necessary for safe, sterile surgery. The spaces of the OR are thus a product not just of surgical technology or medical discourse (Prior 1988), but of the continuing interactions of people and things which have developed in the procedures of modern surgery.

Surgery is an interesting example because it falls mid-way between the 'totalizing' environments which Foucault and Goffman variously chose to explore, and the unrestricted kinds of spaces in which we spend most of our lives. It demonstrates that spaces are not determining, yet can be co-opted to serve particular bodies of knowledge, power interests or subjectivities. To explore the relevance of spatiality to the latter, I shall now consider the ways in which spaces affect older adults living in residential accommodation.

Space and Subjectivity

During field-work in Australia in 1997, I talked to older adults living in 'hostel' and nursing home accommodation. While space was not a central concern in these interviews, it was regularly mentioned by respondents. Given the physical context of these interviews, usually in the rooms of the residents, spatiality was often on the minds of interviewee and myself as we talked together. A frequent theme in these discussions was how issues of space had been a factor in leading to a decision to move into residential accommodation.

> *Mrs R:* I was on my own in the big house and then I noticed – we'd seen this little cottage homes place near the shopping centre, so I sold my big home and I went down there to live and I was there for four and a half years or so. ... I had the opportunity when I sold my place to buy this place down here, and that's what I did, because it was nearer for me and, you know, easier. Of course they used to cut all the lawns and things like that and do all the hard work around the place. ... I had had a bit of a bad back so that's how I came to come down here because the doctor didn't want me on my own.

> *Mrs C:* I told [son] to go and look for a place. I said, 'You go and look for a place' and he knew which places to look for because he works in Medicare so he got this one, which I'm glad he has. Because a lot of

them are three storeys high. You see, I've got my scooter [electric chair], I can scoot around in because I can't walk any distance. No, it suits me just nice.

The change from a house to a relatively small apartment was experienced in a variety of ways. For some respondents it seemed limiting.

Mrs S: This week I haven't felt good at all. The man across has been getting the paper for me because I just haven't been able to get to the foyer to get it. And that annoys me. That really bugs me. I hate staying in this room. I mean, I like my room and I like my view but you can't stay in four walls all day. So I like to get out somewhere at least twice a day, to sit somewhere different or to sit outside for an hour or so.

Mr L: ... if you had more than one room. So you could get away from one another for a while with two separate rooms or something like that. At least you could have a bit of time to yourself.

For others, it was a liberation from the constraints which they had found in their old houses.

Mrs E: I can do what I want to do here. I haven't very much room but I manage fine. I manage really well and I don't have to dust all those things up there. Somebody else does that. ... I had much more furniture than this, much more. But there just wasn't room for it and it's quite hard – I can't get to what's up in that top cupboard. I have to get someone to do that for me.

Mrs H: ... we looked around several places but this was the one I liked best because it had no lifts, no stairs. It was practically on all level ground. And it suited me fine because of my leg. And that's how I came to get here, and I adore it here. I wouldn't be anywhere else. It was the best move I ever made.

Some of the respondents were keen to point out how the advantages of manageable accommodation outweighed the restrictions.

Mrs C: Oh, there's a lot of difference because you're getting waited on here and all that sort of thing. Because I can't get and do things like I used to and all that so, it's not like your own home, you know. Any place isn't; it's not your own place and you can go and do what you want to do and get around, but, you know, in the circumstances there's nothing wrong with it. You just know that you can't do and that's it. So there's nothing wrong with it down here. I'm quite happy here. I've got used to it, you know.

Mr K: I spoke to one of the nurses and she came back and said: 'He's our new ambassador', because I've taken three people around to show them the place. And it's worth doing that because they come in here and they say: 'Gee, what a wonderful room! When you look at it for two people, it's not a box is it?' You look in the bathroom, it's as big as this bedroom. *Mrs K:* My sister-in-law said: 'Isn't the bathroom huge?' I said: 'Yes, father goes for a swim every morning.'

More generally, space and mobility was something which some respondents regretted losing as they grew older. For these respondents, confinement seemed one of the worst features of ageing.

Mr M: ... we used to go dancing on a Saturday night; we used to go to football on a Sunday afternoon. I used to go round to her place and take her to lunch down the hotel and then go to dinner myself at the hotel at five bucks each. ... And I'm a member of the Riverland Classic Car Club. I have two motorcycles, one's a '37 Triumph, the other one's a '47 Norton which I used to go on outings with them. ... That was most of my life like that.

Mr W: There's plenty of activities here that I can't join in because I'm blind. I can't see but they say, 'come in and have a look' but it's no good me going. ... The son's in ____ and the daughter's up at ____ I don't go up there very often because I've got to catch the bus and I can't catch the bus now because ... I could get a free pass on the bus being blind but it's no good me catching the bus because I can't see. I've got to have an attendant all the time. ... No, my advice to anybody is if you can, stay in your own place.

This last respondent, who had delivered newspapers for a living earlier in his life, considered his mobility to be paramount to sustaining his sense of self. He had a regular routine of walking the streets around the home.

Mr W: Well, I get up at quarter to five, have my shower and get dressed and that and then I go out for a walk. I went out on the streets for half past five. I have the street lights to show me the way and I've done 22 streets this morning before I came in and had breakfast. ... then I go walking again. I done 42 streets all told. By the end of June I'll have done 5,000 streets. ... when I'm out walking, I can't see, but I always say good morning, and they always respond. And even the school kids, they will say good morning, you know. And that gives you a sort of a warm glow when kids are wishing you good morning.

Taking responsibility for the space where they lived was also a means of retaining self-respect. When I visited Mr K, he had been cutting back a hedge opposite his window.

Mr K: I've cleaned up the front here. Out here it was a disgrace but I think what's happened is that the people in here are not capable of looking after those window boxes. You are expected to look after the outside as well as the inside without being told. That means you put the broom on; you clean the little pots on both sides of you and keep it looking nice. You're not told to. But you can see when we came here they were neglected.

Mr and Mrs A shared a small apartment which contrasted with the large property where they had lived previously. But the space reduction also signified a loss of autonomy.

Mrs A: ... you lose your responsibility when you come into these sort of places and you haven't got that, you know, to be responsible for – the shopping, the cleaning, the cooking and everything. When you come in here, you haven't got that responsibility and it's not good to have no responsibility for anything. And that is very hard.

These extracts suggest that space may be invested with all sorts of meanings: as limitation or liberation, as supplying a point to daily life, or a sense of selfhood. Unlike the materials considered earlier around the use of space in the OR, here spaces are multiple and not formalized: in many cases, the spaces people inhabited were of their own choosing, and extended (as in the cases of Mr K and Mr W) into the environment beyond the residential housing. We can see the same threads however, of space as something which does not itself constrain, but which acts as a cue to ways of thinking about the world and the body. For Mrs C and Mrs S, the restrictions on space were metonymic for the restrictions of ageing itself. Mr K measured his life against what he could do. He had told me that 'when you're 40, you're 40 per cent in the grave ... you don't realize when you're

dead'. He could hardly bear to be inside for the
.ew.

reduced space available liberated them from anxiety
.cidents. Mrs H was critical of older people who refused
ial accommodation and did not accept the loss of inde-
she saw as an inevitable feature of growing old. For these
ise of self was not reduced by the limits of physical space.

I in.   d the data from these two studies to suggest that space
impinges upon people's activities and subjectivities in ways which cannot
be reduced to physical properties. Unlike the totalizing spaces described in
some analyses, space is a flexible resource whose constraint is dependent
less on absolute materiality than upon the ways in which it is thought. In
the following section, I shall explore another feature of the world which is
often considered to be part of the physical universe: time.

Time and Power

Sociologists from Weber and Marx to the present have acknowledged –
directly or indirectly – the importance of time and timing to modernity
and modernism. Weber (1971: 60ff) saw the history of modern capitalism
as a history of rationalism and of rationalization, and rationalization is
about the organization of people and objects in space and time. The calculability of ends and means supplies a *formal rationality* to modern
organization, of which calculation of time and the associated economic
cost is one part (Brubaker 1984: 36, Fox 1991: 714–17). In Marxist theory,
capitalism commodified labour power, which is bought and sold at rates
standardized according to hours worked.

Within industrial capitalism, this rationalization can be seen clearly,
with such figures as Henry Ford and Frederick Taylor prominent in the
space/time structuring of workplaces. Taylor's contribution was analytical:
he broke down productive tasks into component parts, leading to time-
saving increases in productivity as workers concentrated on a part rather
than a whole. Ford's contribution was complementary: he devised the
production line upon which Taylorized production was to be achieved
(Morgan 1997: 30). Together they made possible the rationalization of the
industrial labour process, and the implementation of higher production
targets based on increased speed of working. Workers on an automated
production line were required to work at the speed of the line, breaks were
institutionalized, and the workers were subjected to managerial regimes
and systems of rules governing how and when they might begin and finish
work (ibid.: 31).

For the individual worker this has led to a routinization of life (Adam 1990: 106–7). Work began each morning when the factory siren sounded, and workers had to 'clock-in' and 'clock-out' to confirm their hours of working. The factory system was based on the co-ordination in time and space of large numbers of workers (Helman 1992: 3). Holidays were no longer flexible: they had to be taken to suit the factory's organization. In the north of England, whole towns and cities closed down for two weeks every year while the employees took vacations. Because the production-line system was threatened by casual absences by staff, absenteeism became a problem for the managers of industry, and systems were implemented to regulate absence due to real or feigned sickness. Taking time off from work on the pretence of sickness remains a means of resistance open to workers, and a problem for industry and economies. As Starkey puts it, time 'is always too short for management and too long for labour' (Starkey 1992: 94). Finally, the life course itself was organized to meet the needs of industry. Workers were recruited in their teenage years, and worked until retirement age, which in the UK – until recently – was set at 65 for men and 60 for women. The traditional retirement present after a lifetime of work was – ironically – a clock or a gold watch, upon which the retired person could watch the seconds of their remaining life tick away.

Some of these regimes of industrial capitalism have been modified, particularly in relation to production lines. Flexible specialization (post-Fordism or Fujitsuism) has sought to involve workers much more fully in production, seeing a product through from beginning to end rather than simply working on one constituent part, over and over (Morgan 1997). Analysis of such innovations as just-in-time and total quality management which derive from post-Fordism have applied understandings of time deriving from Foucault, in which time is seen as a mechanism of control through surveillance (Sewell and Wilkinson 1992). Foucault's studies of disciplinary regimes often recognize the part played by time: from the meting out of carefully calculated sentences to prisoners (Foucault 1979: 107–8), the timetabling of work, military drill and education (ibid.: 149–56) to the years of study required for medical training (Foucault 1976: 81).

These perspectives focus our attention on the relevance of time and timing in the control of individuals, on the imposition of culture on unruly nature. Both seem relevant to the study of health care. The modern health-care system has many attributes of the production line, with the sick person as the raw material and the healed person as the product. Hospitals are overseen by faceless bureaucrats or domineering senior doctors: they are rigidly hierarchical, impersonal and unresponsive to innovation. Particularly in nursing, staff learn sets of actions to be taken in different circumstances: these protocols or 'care plans' determine the treatment a patient receives (Fox 1995a). For patients, experiences of health care – in clinics, wards or residential care – are of routinization and of regimes which reduce the possibility for action (Fox 1992, Strong 1978, Zerubavel 1979). For those with an illness requiring extended hospitalization, their whole lives are routinized by contacts with caring institutions and professions (Roth 1963, Goffman 1968, Kleinman 1988: 181).

However, where there is power there is resistance to it, so it may be that we can identify time, timing and temporality as a potential site of a struggle, between forces of control and other forces resistant to that control. The rationalizations of modernity seek a linear, absolute time, but this search may be a consequence of its impossibility: of the relativity of time, between actors and between contexts and points of view. Rationalization is an exercise of power, made significant only because of the resistances which refuse to submit.

If this is so, then rationalization also contains the seeds of its own destruction. The history of efforts (such as Fordism, post-Fordism and just-in-time management) to establish order is posited upon the resistances of others who would disrupt this and reimpose chaos. Time in modernism is a currency for transaction (Adam 1990: 114, Helman 1992: 40), but not just for those engaged in the economic co-ordination of capitalist society. Strauss *et al.* (1985: 282) suggest that time is integral to the social organization of many aspects of life including health and health care, but that this order is negotiated and flexible. Similarly, in her study of professionalization, Coffey (1994) describes how time

> ... forms a part of the process of negotiation and interaction, which newcomers to an occupational or organizational setting engage in. ... The temporal nature of professional commitment, and the relationship between the individual and the organization recognizes the potential commodification of time in the workplace setting. Time can be bought, sold or given in pursuit of organizational commitment. (Coffey 1994: 954–5)

For professionals, Coffey argues, time is a currency at a symbolic as well as a strictly material level, something which is constitutive of what Bourdieu calls *habitus* (Bourdieu 1990: 9–10). We might add that time is something which is bought, sold and bartered in all aspects of life – not only work – from birth to the grave. Because it can be traded (not only in a strict economic sense, but also symbolically), the economy of time may be not only a tool for those who seek power and control, but also an adjunct for a campaign of resistance to rationalization.

Once again I am going to look at data from the studies of surgical organization and the experiences of older adults to explore these ideas about the use of time in the context of health care. I will both document the controlling aspect of time, and consider how the passage of time can sometimes be a tool or resource for resisting or refusing power, a commodity which can be negotiated, appropriated or 'wasted'. So I will focus not only on the rationalizations and routines of health and care (Roth 1963, Zerubavel 1979), but also on the events where time seems to break free from control and offers possibilities for challenges by the subjects of rationalization.

I Time Flies: the Routines of Day Case Surgery

During my field-work at General Hospital, I observed the organization of surgical services in a range of services. One of these was day case surgery (DCS), then a new departure at the hospital, though now common practice for a wide range of surgical procedures.

Timing is central to day surgery: indeed it is the feature which defines it. By its very nature, day surgery emphasizes the operation, and by limiting the hospital stay to a few hours before and after the procedure, de-emphasizes these periods. DCS is part of a drive for efficient use of resources, pushing as many patients through the hospital as can physically be included on a day-long surgical list, avoiding at least one limitation: that imposed by availability of beds. A patient on a DCS list may have been discharged before the list upon which she or he was included has even been completed, while a surgeon may see a patient only when unconscious upon the table, particularly if the pre-operative examination is conducted by a junior. As such, it is a case study of how time can dominate a process, reducing it to the equivalent of a production line.

The following data was collected during a day spent on the DCS Unit at General Hospital, some four months after it opened. The unit was converted from existing buildings and comprised a small reception area, a Nightingale-style ward with space for 15 trolley-beds which could be wheeled directly to the operating theatre (OR) and, towards the far end of the unit, offices, rest room, sluice etc. A door at the far end (for staff use only) led to the main hospital concourse, and was located virtually opposite the entrance to the OR. Each bed area was provided with an oxygen line and suction, and could be curtained off. The unit opened each working day at 8 a.m. and normally closed at 6 p.m. when the last patient of the day was discharged. Typical daily staffing comprised the clinical manager Dr F (an anaesthetist and part-time manager), a receptionist, a ward sister, a staff nurse, an enrolled nurse (SEN) and two nursing auxiliaries. Patients were processed by the receptionist on arrival, and waited in a small room next to reception until nursing staff were ready to allocate them to a trolley.

Time

8.07 a.m.   The first patient arrives and, having been seen by the receptionist, is taken by a nurse to trolley-bed 8. She sits on the edge of the bed, the curtains are drawn and the patient undresses and puts on a surgical gown.

8.13 a.m.   As patients arrive they are asked to wait in the waiting area. They are then called back to reception, and checked in by the ward sister. A patient has arrived unexpectedly, having not confirmed his appointment.
Sister: 'Sorry, we had a place, but it's been filled. You'll have to come back next week.'

8.17 a.m.   Patients in beds 9 and 4, accompanied by parents.

8.25 a.m.   House doctor arrives, checks list, and goes to bed 2, now occupied.

8.26 a.m.   Beds 3 and 10 occupied. A rush of patients arriving means a wait before being taken to their trolleys.

8.30 a.m.   Bed 4 patient is brought from the waiting area. Patients are scheduled for phased arrival up to 9.00 a.m., but a wait of 15 minutes has developed as patients are processed into their places.
Patients are ticked off on a board at the nursing station, and details of transport home noted: 'Mother'; 'Mum staying'; 'We will phone'. Plastic identity bracelets are attached to patients once in bed.

8.32 a.m.   Anaesthetist Dr R sees patient in bed 6. 'How about if we don't put you to sleep?' Dr R sees the patients in turn, some are given pre-medication, depending on the procedure, and the history of the patient.

8.35 a.m.   Bed 5 patient arrives.

8.52 a.m.   Porter arrives, and wheels the patient in Bed 1 to the OR. Manager Dr F arrives and confers with ward sister. The unit is servicing three lists today: an oral list (beds 1–5) in the designated OR, an orthopaedic list in theatre S (beds 6–8), and a plastic list (10–11). Patients are taken to the three theatres when called.

9.00 a.m.   Surgical lists begin in the various ORs.

10.15 a.m.   Patient 1 returns from recovery. The nursing staff are trained in recovery, and are detailed to ensure the patients are ready to leave at the appropriate time.

Sister: 'We try not to give strong post-operative medication, and not necessarily a pre-med. We need to ensure a patient can get here and back without driving. If we aren't happy that a patient has recovered, or there is a problem with getting him home then they may have to be kept in.'

Researcher: 'How often does this happen?'

Auxiliary: (looking through records) 'Eight times this month, 26 (in the past four months).'

12.30 p.m.   Patient in bed 2 discharged. Relatives of other patients are waiting for decisions on discharge, which are made by ward sister, after consultation with clinicians.

12.40 p.m.   Sister, SEN and one auxiliary go to lunch, leaving staff nurse in control of unit.

1.05 p.m.   The oral surgery list is complete. Mr P comes to the unit, and leaves some instructions with the staff nurse. Patients are discharged throughout the afternoon.

4.40 p.m.   Unit closes.

The comings and goings of patients continued throughout the day. The highly co-ordinated activities in the DCS Unit influence the timing of surgery in the various ORs, with an emphasis on moving patients swiftly and efficiently through surgery, as the following extract from field notes in the OR that day demonstrates.

Time

11.05 a.m.   Patient is brought into the OR, having been anaesthetised after a 30-minute wait in the anaesthetic room. The operation begins: the removal of wires following a road traffic accident two weeks previously.

11.15 a.m.   Anaesthetist Dr R: (to surgeon) 'Is it time for the next patient?' (i.e. to have the porter bring the next patient to the anaesthetic room).

Surgeon Mr P: 'No.'

11.35 a.m.   Jaw wires removed, Mr P begins on the wires which have been inserted through the eyebrows. These do not come out so easily, and there is haemorrhaging, which causes adverse commentary from the anaesthetist, and apologies from Mr P.

11.45 a.m.   First wire removed.
11.50 a.m.   Second wire removed. Mr P: 'OK, we're sewing up now'.
11.52 a.m.   Mr P: (to anaesthetist) 'OK.' Dr R sends for next patient.
11.56 a.m.   First patient is taken to recovery. Dr R goes to the anaesthetic
             room and induces the next patient.

As pre-operative patients in the unit are replaced with those recovering post-operatively, the mood of frenetic activity is replaced by a much more tranquil routine of care, discharge and administrative duties. If all goes according to plan surgically, the processing of patients throughout the day means none will have to be admitted to the hospital (entailing removal to a different ward). This ethnographic extract suggest an efficient 'well-oiled machine' in which staff achieve a smooth production line of patients successfully treated. As such it might be considered to epitomize the modernist rationalizations discussed earlier. This is reflected in the comment made by Dr F, the clinical manager, to the researcher nine months previously. For him, any problems were managerial.

> *Dr F:* Developing day surgery is a matter of resourcing and logistics. It does entail a change in surgical practice but not so much in terms of technique as in management. The research which is needed concerns feasibility – what kind of surgery might be done ... ward design and operational policy.

The economic rationalism of the production line of DCS required all involved – patients and staff – to accept the control which the regime entailed. This had negative consequences for care and for job satisfaction, as these staff members noted.

> *Staff Nurse:* We don't see the patients ill, and then getting better. It's dissatisfying working here.
> *Nurse Auxiliary:* There's no time to fill out a care plan for an individual patient, so we can't give them appropriate care.
> *Staff Nurse:* We had a man yesterday and because I hadn't got to know him even for a day, I couldn't give him the reassurance before the operation. I felt like a shop-keeper or a hairdresser. I'm looking forward to (leaving).

In this first case, I have documented the use of time as a managerial technique to enhance efficiency. It is – in fact – a good example of 'just-in-time' management, with no slack in the system, and the need for all sections of an organization to work in tandem. Here time is a mechanism or a technology for control: workers must work at the speed of the organization, and with a defined workload that must be completed in a day (it is highly inconvenient to all concerned if DCS patients have to stay overnight in hospital) they know they have little choice but to keep the patients moving as if on a production line.

In chapter 1, I drew upon some data from another surgical case study, concerning surgeons' ward rounds and discussions of discharge. I want to return to this data to illustrate another economy in which time is important, not only as the medium within which the negotiations take place, but also as the currency to be negotiated.

II Buying Time: Patients, Surgeons and Discharge Dates

For patients whose surgery cannot be conducted on a day case basis, the inevitable consequence of undergoing surgery is a stay in hospital postoperatively, to overcome the physiological affect of prolonged anaesthesia and to confirm that wound healing has begun, free from the complications of infection. With recent innovations such as 'key-hole' surgery and with post-operative support available in the community, stays are now much shorter following many surgical procedures, but the period between an operation and discharge is still a time in which both patients and surgeons must 'wait for nature to take its course'. When I conducted this field-work, most surgical patients would expect at least five days on the ward post-operatively.

The agendas of patient and surgeon might be quite different during this period. For surgeons, time is needed to assess the recovery of the patient, while for the patient, a return to home and life beyond the constraints of hospital are a priority. In such circumstances, time-scales may also differ. From the surgeon's perspective, the time between post-operative visits to a patient may pass quickly; for the patient, two or three days between ward rounds can seem an eternity. So perhaps it is unsurprising that issues around time are raised in many of these encounters, as the surgical ward round comes to be seen as an event crucial in determining a patient's immediate future. The first extract in this section – taken from a Friday morning round – was typical of a first post-operative visit, and indicates the differing agendas of surgeon and patient.

(Patient C has undergone surgery to remove an ovarian cyst. Surgeon Mrs A is seeing her 24 hours later.)
Surgeon A: Hallo Mrs C, we have sorted out your problem for you. Let us have a look at your tummy.

(Staff nurse and junior doctor pull curtains around, Mrs C is laid flat, and the dressing is removed.)
Surgeon A: Yes, that's OK. You will not have much of a scar there.
Patient C: Thank you. When can I go home?
Surgeon A: We'll see you on Monday. (to nurse) Can I have a (type of dressing) please.

Even for patients who did not expect an immediate discharge, the ward round punctuated the monotony of hospital life. Furthermore, it was an occasion which could give indications about the future, about what a patient might expect. Patient N had had major surgery for carcinoma of the bowel. She prepared herself for the twice-weekly ward round, applying make-up and sitting up in bed to await surgeon Mr D, who perceived her as a problem patient. In the event, she had little chance to negotiate her future, as Mr D whisked himself away.

Surgeon D: How is the ileostomy?
Patient N: It's much better, at least this one works.
Surgeon D: Good.
Patient N: ... (tries to ask a question, but Mr D has moved away and has initiated a conversation with the house doctor).
Surgeon D: We'll see you on Tuesday.

The timetable for discharge is seldom clear-cut, and patients may have no idea whether their condition enables them to leave hospital. But for the surgeon, discharge is often the end of the story, and the decision – once taken – may seem quite casual, perhaps acknowledging that there is unlikely to be dissent given the enthusiasm for most patients to leave.

Surgeon A: (looking at case notes, speaking to house doctor, but across the patient) I think Miss A can go home today. Can we just have a quick look, doctor. (to patient) How are you feeling?
Patient A: OK.
Surgeon A: (looks at the condition of the surgical wound) Well you can go home today, have you someone coming?
Patient A: Yes.
Surgeon A: Well that's OK. Sort that out will you, doctor?

On other occasions, discharge is negotiated, with a patient's home situation weighed up against the risks of discharge. Patient W was an old man who had a major resection for gastric carcinoma.

Surgeon D: Who's going to look after you when you get out?
Patient W: (smiling) You tell me when I can go, and I'll arrange to be looked after.
Surgeon D: (smiling) That's right ... but seriously though?
Patient W: Well, my sister. She's older than me of course, but ...
Surgeon D: Well someone to cook for you?
Patient W: Oh yes, that'll be all right.
Surgeon D: Make a clinic appointment for next Wednesday and you can go home now.
Patient W: When?
Surgeon D: As soon as you can arrange it.
Patient W: (pretends to get out of bed) Well I'll give a ring now. *Thank you.* I'll ring now.

In all these cases, the surgeon seeks to control the interaction. Even though a surgeon cannot – except in extreme circumstances – prevent a patient from discharging her- or himself 'against medical advice', the interactions are framed as if the patient has no say in the matter. Surgeons assert their authority, and their capacity to exercise subtle judgements about discharge is used to sustain this authority.

We can see in this case study a further example of how time is part of a regime of control, but here it is implicated twice. Time is not only the mechanism of control (the infrequent ward round which must be awaited as a crucial determinant of a patient's situation), but it is also in many cases the thing which is being determined (the length of stay in hospital, the expectations for the future following surgery). Time is a resource which is seemingly to be dispensed as largesse by the surgeon. But to 'buy' time, time must first be passed, used up. We are reminded that time is a commodity which can be negotiated, bought and sold.

We might also make a comparison with a prison regime. Here too, the imprisoned must use time to buy time. In England, serving a prison sentence is known as 'doing time'. And it is only when a certain portion of time has been 'done', that there is a possibility that future time may be discounted, for a prisoner to be given a future in which their time is their own rather than that of the prison regime.

In summary, we have seen in these ethnographies of a day case unit and a surgical ward round, two examples of how time is managed and manipulated. In both cases, there seems little room for negotiation. In the first, management used time to maximize efficiency of a service. In the second, time is a commodity to be dispensed by surgeons, and one to be passed passively by patients. However, this is only part of the story, because in different circumstances. time cannot be used so easily as a tool of power or authority. Sometimes time can be manipulated by different groups to their own ends, disrupting routines and introducing the possibility of struggle and resistance.

III Killing Time: the Disruption of Surgical Routines

In addition to the DCS Unit, there were ten surgical operating theatres at General Hospital, and the organization of surgical services was an undertaking involving 120 nursing and auxiliary staff during. day shifts, the provision of supplies ranging from sterile dressings to equipment hardware, and the regulation of the supply of patients to the theatres 24 hours a day. While an operating department manager (ODM) held overall managerial responsibility, each pair of theatres was managed locally by a theatre sister/charge nurse.

My ethnographic study of the routine of the surgical day at General Hospital uncovered constant disruption by a remarkable component of apparent inefficiency and unpredictability. Patients arrived late, or not at all; patients were precipitately removed from lists or substituted by those needing quite different procedures; procedures were not those planned and written into the list; no account of anaesthetic time was made; too many patients were scheduled and lists were unmanageably long requiring staff to work late; instruments were unavailable or not ready at the same time as the patient. In many cases, timing was at the heart of the disruption. The following is an extract from my field notes about a morning in orthopaedic theatre.

Time

10.30 a.m.   The previous patient has been taken to recovery, but although the ward has been contacted to send the next patient, he has not yet arrived.

Anaesthetic Nurse: 'Orthopaedic surgeons are the worst, they arrange things at the last minute, and then they're not organized properly ... they don't communicate. It's probably because so many of them are foreign – they don't understand each other.'

10.45 a.m.   With no patient arriving, the registrar (junior doctor) is sent to look for him. Meanwhile another patient is added to the list, a 16-year-old. But this patient has not been seen by the house doctor, has not been consented, and may not have been starved prior to surgery. The registrar is sent off once again. The original patient is finally found on a different ward.

11.00 a.m.   The registrar returns.

Registrar: 'He had been consented. The staff nurse thought the age of consent was 18 but he's signed himself. His father has been waiting around to sign a consent.'

Surgeon: (to researcher) 'This is the sort of thing that happens. The consultant tells the staff nurse who tells the houseman who forgets or is too busy.'

11.20 a.m.   The patient arrives. He does not want a general anaesthetic and argues with the anaesthetist. He has not received a pre-med and is very upset. He is finally persuaded by the anaesthetist to undergo the procedure.

11.40 a.m.   The patient is wheeled unconscious into the operating theatre.

12.30 a.m.   The final patient on the list is delayed. A call to the ward reveals that half the nursing shift are taking their lunch break and there is no nurse free to accompany the patient to the theatre.

Anaesthetist Dr M: 'This happens every day. They must know it is going to happen, but nothing is done about it.'

After a number of similar experiences, I realized that disruption of routine was the norm in the surgical service at General Hospital. Yet unless coaxed, the delays seemed to be something about which theatre staff preferred not to speak, and there was a general acceptance that an uncertain activity such as surgery could not be regimented by the clock. However, one informant – the anaesthetist Dr J – became an enthusiastic commentator upon the inefficiencies witnessed in theatre. His use of them to define the moral and intellectual superiority of anaesthetists over surgeons is documented elsewhere (Fox 1994). He blamed a variety of people for the delays, from nurses:

Dr J: That call was from the ward – there's no one to come up to theatre with the patient. That usually means that the staff nurse has not planned ahead.

a combination of nurses and patients:

Dr J: Patients are called by letter, and will or will not agree to come in. Sometimes it's difficult to arrange substitutes, but it means you cannot plan with any confidence that the list will be as proposed. Some surgeons anticipate this, and send for more patients than they would expect to get. Then they have too many, and this is irritating if it happens too often. It's a problem for nursing staff, who are very rigid.

and in particular, surgeons:

> *Dr J:* There was absolute chaos here [plastic theatre] yesterday. The list was arranged so that patients were due in theatre hours before they came to hospital. Then in the afternoon, two major cases were put on the list, which meant there was not enough time without keeping staff on after six, and it had to be rearranged, so one case is being done today instead. ... Two or three per cent of patients will have a problem [which makes anaesthesia risky] which cannot be sorted out. The anaesthetist needs to see the patient, but some firms [of surgeons] seem incapable of concocting a list until the morning of the schedule.

Surgeons, on the other hand, found their own culprits, often among the ranks of the lowest in the hierarchy.

> *Surgeon A:* I can't believe it, the man came [to collect a tissue biopsy] and the secretary sent him away. He came all the way from ____ himself and she sent him away.

> *Surgeon B:* Here we are [in the rest-room], all ready to do our work, and we wait on the ministrations of the porter to bring us our work.

Surgeons were defensive about their own culpability in causing delays, and used the excuse of uncertainty to vindicate their actions, for example, in scheduling too many patients on a list.

> *Surgeon Y:* Orthopaedic surgery at General Hospital is on take seven days a week, so there are always emergencies. A list is made up at very short notice. There are patients in the wards, and we decide to add them to a list. People say that they don't have to go on *this* list, but they have to go on *a* list. That's what people forget.

> *Surgeon T:* Yes, there is quite a lot of hanging around, that's the price of being part of a large organization.

They would blame anaesthetists for causing delays between patients, reducing the throughput of patients on a list.

Anaesthetist Dr C: The surgeon does not consider the anaesthesia to be anything other than wasted time, and do not seem to calculate for it when they make up a list. They don't take it into account … Surgeons regard the theatre as their own, they say what will go on. We have to have the patient ready when they want it.

On the other hand, if a patient was induced and ready for surgeons, there was no guarantee the surgeons would similarly be scrubbed and ready. On one occasion observed by the researcher, an anaesthetist had to keep a patient under the anaesthetic for an extended period because the surgeons were still in their office when the patient arrived on the table.

Anaesthetist Dr J: The anaesthetist will arrange a pre-med, either directly, or from theatre via the house officer. Timing is critical, so it is essential to be able to predict the length of surgery.

Overall, the field-work implicated surgeons as the causes of much of the disruption. On one hand, they see uncertainty as a legitimate, if unfortunate, consequence of the surgical enterprise. They perceive last-minute arrangements or changes to lists, changes in procedure, overloading lists and ignoring preparation time as hazards of their uncertain job. For surgeons, those who are to blame are ward nurses and porters, who are not available to ferry patients into the operating theatre, anaesthetists for taking too long in induction and preparation, or patients who do not appear for their surgery. These are all put down to managerial shortcomings.

However, rather than indulging in the same activity of blame-ascription, I want to suggest that we can see the actions of surgeons as a response, a resistance to efforts to impose a managerially-defined regimen upon their work. From a management perspective, control and maintenance of the routines of surgery must be an objective, and this is borne out in the comments of management and theatre sisters.

Operating Department Manager F: The work of the ODM entails a big personnel management task. The day in theatre is 8 a.m. to 5 p.m.; two or three nurses will work a half-day, the others come on the late shift. I make sure that the work gets organized to make the best use of staff. From time to time I look at scheduling, to make efficient use of theatres, and I monitor the amount of emergency operating in sessions.

Clinical Manager Dr M: Emergencies are more of an administrative than a medical emergency. If we are running an efficient unit, we want to run nurses, anaesthetists and equipment all the time. So we fill all the theatres nine to five with elective surgery. If an emergency arises, we need to break into the elective list, and then find extra time for the elective surgery. Surgeons prefer to let the emergencies build up, and then do a list overnight. But that is awful for the patients, because the surgery will be done by on-call surgeons. The alternative is to have three theatres open in the evening – but most of the time two will lie unused.

For operating department manager F, the objective was not simply maximizing throughput, but managing a resource (staff and theatre time) efficiently. She summed up what she perceived as the unreasonable attitudes and behaviours of surgeons.

> *Manager F:* Surgeons are prima donnas, they want theatres to be open longer however long they are open. I keep telling surgeons to control their lists. Recently there was a night with 12 emergency cases. Consultants in thoracic, gynae, neuro and general surgery came in, and they all wanted to operate as quickly as possible. They are only interested in their own patient and what they want to do – they are not interested in their colleagues. They wanted the staff and extra theatres to be available, and it was up to the night sister to decide who went into theatre, in which order. Fortunately she was very experienced, and got it about right, and none of the patients suffered medically. When the surgeons cool off they will realize they were selfish, but since it happened I have had the surgeons on the phone asking me to sort it out so it doesn't happen again. ... Surgeons will try to take advantage day after day, and will use emotional blackmail to try to keep staff on late. One of the surgeons in plastic [theatre] says that if you want to be a theatre nurse you must not have a life of your own. That is old-fashioned!

We might conclude that surgeons were resistant for a reason: not simply because of their contrariness, but because they wished to protect their clinical autonomy: their right to operate how and when they see fit. Managerialism was seen as a threat to this autonomy, attempting to turn 'professionals' into 'employees' (Starkey 1992: 97), and the effort to regiment surgery within specific time constraints was resisted by disrupting those routines. They used the excuse of uncertainty to support their disruption, and because of their position in the hierarchy, management at General Hospital was unable to exercise the control they sought. It was only through management-led initiatives such as day case surgery, where surgeons were effectively bought off with promises of additional operating times, that the efforts to routinize and control actions were successful. I asked an oral surgeon why he had supported day surgery.

> *Surgeon P:* I did not have the all-day list which I wanted. Now with the day case unit I will have. I had to cancel a clinic but the day case unit has given me the opportunity to get what I wanted. I can mix day case and non-day case patients, it does not matter one iota ...

In summary, we can see that once again time is a resource. But in this case study, there was a more even battle of authorities, and time became the medium of a struggle. Time was something to be fought over, a territory to be won or lost like any other. Management sought to impose routines, surgeons resisted these and asserted their clinical autonomy. In the confines of the OR, they could act much as they pleased, resorting to claims of clinical judgement when the smooth operation of the theatre was disrupted by their activities. Management fought back with new strategies to impose order. The implementation of day surgery, with its set routines and production-line model of surgery, was won by offering something (a change of timing, as it happens) in return. Once again, time can be seen as a commodity which is bought, sold and struggled over.

IV Time on their Hands: Growing Old in Australia

Is it possible then to have too much time? To explore this aspect, I shall draw on more data from the study of older Australians' experiences of growing old. Recalling the situation of the people awaiting discharge from surgery, it was argued that they were having to spend time (recuperating) to buy time (their lives beyond the hospital). For the old people in this study, there was not a similar bargain to be made. They were using their time (their lives in the residential homes) but there is nothing beyond that this time can purchase. If the quality of their present time-spending was not satisfactory, there was nothing in recompense. Time now becomes something which is spent with little to show for it.

> *Mr M:* Time is a big factor in a place like this when you're an invalid.
> *Researcher:* So time is something which you've got quite a lot of?
> *Mr M:* Yes we have. I go asking 'what day is it today?' because when you're not working you don't realize what day it is.

> *Researcher:* Is there any aspect of your life which you miss?
> *Mrs G:* I had more work to do. I kept busier and no time to think how sad you were when you lost anybody.

Time was a resource only if it was filled: when there was nothing to fill it, it constrained. The abundance of time threatened to overwhelm, and had to be resisted.

Mrs S: I hate staying in this room. I mean I like this room and I like my view but you can't stay in four walls all day. So I like to get out somewhere at least twice a day, to sit somewhere different or to sit outside for an hour or so. You must keep the old mind working, that's what I think anyway.

Mrs H: I sometimes have visitors. And there's often things here that I can go to during the afternoon and mostly I just sit around here like this and wait for lunch time. And then I go down to lunch and if there's anything on, I stay down and see it out. ... It's something to do at any rate, keeps your mind occupied.

Empty time was to be avoided, as without something to fill the time, life would deteriorate. Keeping busy becomes an end in itself.

Mr K: Activity, not to sit here and decay. ... I've had (cancer) since 1981 and fighting it all the time. And that's why the activity comes in. The activity has kept me going ... I would put in 30 hours in a week but I had book work, mental work to do, and it wasn't hard because if you didn't feel like doing it, you're not forced to do it.

Mr M: Nice surroundings I'd say and things to do. Occupational therapy you could say it would be.

As time became emptier, life was duller, with little to fill the time between events, and nothing to look forward to.

Mrs S: I don't think about the future very much. We've just got to live a quiet life and we know quite a few of the people around. There's different things we can do. We can read although I'm getting to the stage where I can't read, and that's a bit of a disappointment because I thought I would always be able to read. I think I live quite a dull life now, but the family are good.

Mr W: All I've got is my walking.

In this chapter I have argued that time is a resource, and as such is something which may be the site of struggle and resistance. But it is not time itself which is the objective to be obtained, but the things with which one may fill it (Derrida 1993: 3). So perhaps it is the potentiality that time offers which makes it so desirable to have at one's disposal. It is like money, of little use in its own right, but highly desirable because it is capable of being traded for virtually anything. Yet, in this final case, we have seen a situation in which time is no longer a currency. Rather than being a scarce commodity, it is in abundance, and rather than being a resource, it is an encumbrance: it is a coinage which is no longer recognized. The lack of things to fill the time available makes a mockery of it and its passage, and empty time comes to be feared as something which will lead to introversion, loneliness and depression. Time now becomes the enemy of the self, not the means for self-actualization. Ironically, the comments reported here were offered against a backcloth of a staffing shortage, in which time was in very short supply for those working in the homes: elsewhere in the interviews, many residents commented about how *little* time staff had for them.

Chronicity and Health

Time is central to the way in which humans perceive the world, and in the modern period, the principal way of thinking about time has been as a resource which has an economic value attached to it (Adam 1995: 91). Time does not, however, have a single meaning, and its significance varies – depending upon the situation and upon the point of view of those involved. From what has preceded, we might identify:

- Time as a unit of economic value (the hours worked to make money, the time taken to make a commodity)
- Time as a resource to be managed, manipulated or controlled by organizational systems to maximize achievement of an objective, and thus also available as a site of resistance
- Time as something to be bartered, bought, sold or given away by individuals
- Time as something to be filled

In all of these categories, time is not a natural phenomenon, rather it is a cultural attribute which is constructed and utilized socially, and may have a variety of meanings. This proposition that time is cultural through and through requires some exploration, as it contradicts some other theorizations of time.

Helman (1992) uses Hall's (1984) distinction between *monochronic* and *polychronic* times to explore the impact of time and timing regimes on health and illness. It is argued that – in the modern period (which began with the Enlightenment around 1800) – the West has been dominated with a *mono-chronic* notion of time. Time is seen as linear, an absolute within a Newtonian universe against which lives are measured and passed (Adam 1990: 52, Game 1991: 93). Monochronic time is 'public' time, also 'male' time (Helman 1992: 38), while polychronic time is associated with private spheres such as the home, and often with 'female' orientations towards people and relationships (ibid). Elsewhere, Helman suggests that the latter is

> the more human, qualitative time, the time of people, and not of punc-tuality – and the time of doing things for them, and with them. Here tasks are completed only 'when the time is right' and not before. So food must be prepared for the palate or for friends, and not just for the clock – and social talk and human warmth are more important than diaries and appointments. (Helman 1991: 130–1)

Helman's argument is tinged with romanticism, especially when he speaks of polychronic time as enabling a return to the 'timeless cycles of the ancient myths' (Helman 1991: 139). For him, time has been subverted and we need to rescue ourselves from monochronic (cultural) time if we are to avoid some of the risks to health of the modern world such as stress-related heart disease (Helman 1992: 43).

The opposition of cultural time and natural time is also to be seen in Adam's work. In an effort to demonstrate the mutual implication of the notions of time and health, Adam (1992) argues that we live both in the world of clock time and in the rhythmic time of nature and the body. The latter, which she calls 'temporal time' (Adam 1992: 161) is not like linear time, but is based on the 'present-creating-becoming' (ibid.: 163) which is a feature of life. Unfortunately Adam's analysis only works if one accepts a realist perspective on knowledge, in which we have the capacity to use our reason to see beyond linear time to this underlying temporal time. Even if our bodies somehow 'know' the truth of these natural rhythms physiologically (ibid.: 155), Adam argues her case not in terms of 'gut feeling' but rationally and intellectually, using clock time as the measure against which the rhythms of temporal time are found to be incommen-surate (for example that sometimes it seems that time 'flies by' and at other times dawdles along). Yet if clock time is a social construction, what can be the status of the entities which it enables us to perceive? Her addi-tional argument that temporal time has been discerned as a 'law of nature' by physicists (ibid.: 162) fails to acknowledge that such concepts are elements in theory, not 'hard facts'.

We can make some propositions concerning a time which is social through and through. For example, a distinction can be made between institutional time and personal time. For the institution, time may be a commodity in short supply, and control of it may be both a source of power and a means to attain power and authority. From a personal point of view, time may not have the same value as it has for an organization, and sometimes one block of time may be traded for another which is seen as more valuable. As Adam (1990: 114) has also noted, in some instances, the time at one's disposal is highly valuable (for instance, a surgeon's time), in others, it may be virtually worthless (for instance, the time of an unskilled or retired person). This value, however, is not only a 'market value' but also a personal value: for someone who has a lot to cram into limited time, the personal value of time cannot be reflected in its 'market value'. Coffey suggests (1994: 955) that this highlights the tensions between personal autonomy and organizational control. I would add that it is also a tool which renders humans capable of resisting power: time may be manipulat_d precisely *because* it can have various meanings and values for different participants in a setting.

Health and health care are inextricably tied up with issues of human finitude: for humans, time is by necessity limited. In a capitalist economy, this limited time is appropriated by its commodification as work, and time often becomes equated with money. But this is only part of the story, as I have tried to demonstrate. Time is commodified in other ways as well, and can be bought, sold and given according to different regimes. In the operating theatre, it is used as a means to control or resist power. On the wards, it is bartered against future time. In the old people's home, it is a commodity with little value, and can become an encumbrance rather than a resource.

Chronicity is deeply implicated in constructing a subjectivity, and this is particularly important in issues of health and illness. Chronic illness is defined by its relation with time, yet, as Kleinman points out, this is an entirely social, and therefore contingent, process.

Chronicity ... is the outcome of lives lived under constraining circumstances with particular relationships to other people. Chronicity is created in part out of negative expectations that come to be shared in face-to-face interactions – expectations that fetter our dreams and sting and choke our sense of self. Patients learn to act as chronic cases; family members and care givers learn to treat patients in keeping with this view. (Kleinman 1988: 180)

We collude (Kleinman goes on) in building walls and tearing down bridges to new possibilities. People are defined as uni-dimensional – patients, the disabled, the life-threatened – as if this were all they are. We trap people in a frontier zone, where they wander confused and desperate to return to their native land (ibid.: 180–1).

Challenging these limiting ways of thinking means rejecting and refusing the power of time and chronicity. As we study and research health and health care, we need to address how time is used, and the differing meanings it may have for different participants in the setting. If modernism has emphasized the commodification of time, it has concomitantly established it as something to be contested and thus as a site for alternative claims to 'truth' (Derrida 1976: 12). Resistance – in the context of time, as with other resources – may be *negative* (a refusal or rejection such as an industrial strike in which workers refuse to sell their time to an employer), or *positive*: a breaking-free from constraining notions of time as currency or something to be feared for its emptiness. The humanities have supplied examples of such creative rethinkings of time: from Proust's experiment in memory and reflexivity (*A la recherche du temps perdu: In Search of Lost Time*) to Freud's 'talking cure' of fabricated pasts (Game 1991: 90ff). All these times are social, and that – not recourse to a return to 'natural time' – is what makes resistance possible.

Concluding Remarks

In this chapter I have taken the two dimensions of space and time and explored the context-dependence of these features of life for people involved in issues around health and illness. I hope that I have shown that they may be implicated in the mediation of power and control, and that spatiality and temporality are resources to be drawn on in constituting subjectivity or sense-of-self. My analysis has also, I hope, indicated that if space and time are sites of power, they may also be sites of resistance: the theme of the second part of this book. For social science explorations of health and care, this suggests a double agenda. First, to examine aspects of modernist organization and experience of health and care to uncover how space and time are used not only as a technique of power, but also as a strategy for resistance. Second (and this task has hardly begun), to explore how resisting modernity's spatiality and temporality might shape human growth and self-actualization, to move *beyond* health.

3
The Ethics and Politics of Caring

What does it mean to care? And what is the significance of being a caregiver or a recipient of care? In this chapter, I shall explore the relevance of this category of human activity for the project of understanding health, illness and what it means to move beyond such formulations, using theoretical perspectives from various postmodern writers including Foucault, Derrida and Cixous. Under the general banner of postmodernism, various writings have espoused an ethics that (perhaps paradoxically) offers possibilities for engagement with others, overcoming the moral relativism of modernism (Bauman 1989, 1993b, Caputo 1993, Fox 1993a, White 1991) and reintroducing a concern with the politics of the social world. By looking at issues in care, this chapter supplies important ethical and political agendas for the project which this book develops.

Within the social sciences, 'care' is paradoxical. On one hand, it is based in intimate and human relations which value giving, love and concern. On the other, it is a set of practices – and theories about those practices – which are codified by the 'caring professions' as an occupation and the basis for disciplinary power and authority (Gardner 1992). As Thomas (1993: 649) also points out, care entails both the emotional 'caring about someone' and the more instrumental 'caring for a person'. 'Care' is a growth area for theory at the present time, and careers in care professions and in research and academic life are being forged from the disciplinary work of care theorists: the fabrication of what I shall call *care-as-discipline* or the *vigil* of care. The *vigil* is about power, and following Foucault (1980a), this power is intricately associated with knowledge, in this case the knowledge deriving from theories of care. The unfortunate subjects of this power/knowledge work are the recipients of care-as-discipline.

Within such theorizing, we may weigh the sociological literature: the social sciences have devoted substantial time and space to explorations of the character of 'caring' (Graham 1991, James 1989, Marsden and Abrams 1987, Thomas 1993), the institutions by which it has become part of modern culture (Foucault 1976, 1986, Rose 1989, Summers 1979), and to our ambivalence about some of the achievements of the caring society (de Swaan 1990, Goffman 1968, Maseide 1991, Roberts 1985). As I write these words, policy-makers in the United Kingdom have concluded that 'care in the community' (one of the most theorized aspects of the welfare system) has failed many people in need of care. We may expect a new flood of theory and policy in response to such claims.

So the first task of this chapter is to understand the impact of this theorizing of a *vigil* of care. But it is also about the ways in which it is possible to resist the *vigil* of care, and its continued opposition by a different kind of 'care' which celebrates difference and is mediated by love, generosity, trust and delight – a *gift* of care. I will look at theories of gifts later in the chapter, in particular the analyses deriving from Derrida and the feminist Cixous. The latter's notion of the *gift* opposes interpersonal relations within caring which are based in generosity and a celebration of difference with the possessive, controlling 'care-as-discipline'. Finally, this chapter is about the implications of such a different care for professional carers and those for whom they care.

I cannot hope to explore the entire range of systems of thought by which care, carers and those who are cared for are constructed. As has already been indicated, many studies have documented some of these elements: the gendering of the social relations of care, the work entailed in managing emotions, and the dependency and transference which may underpin caring. Rather than recapitulating these themes, in examining the vigil of care I shall focus specifically upon the fabrication of caring as a professional activity. Before that, I should like to make three points which will orient the reader towards some issues which the subsequent analysis raises.

1. The first point concerns the theoretical underpinning of post-structuralism, and in particular positions concerning power and subjectivity. Were the postulated opposition of 'care-as-discipline' and 'care-as-gift' to be couched in an essentialist or foundationalist framework, analysis would perhaps suggest how empowerment (individual or collective) could overcome institutional control, oppression or domination. A post-structuralist framework does not offer so straightforward a resolution, for the simple reason that from this perspective, there is no longer an essential subject. Subjectivity is an outcome of power/knowledge: and both discourse (care-as-discipline) and resistance to it (care-as-*gift*) operate

in the same domain, namely that of language. This means that the mechanism of the *vigil's* disciplinary power is not situated outside the care setting – in policy or institutions or educational establishments (although these are often the places where systems of thought are codified) – but in the everyday practice of care, in the contact between carer and cared-for. But it is also within these contacts that the possibilities of resistance are to be found: documenting the *vigil* of care suggests how it may be resisted.

2. At a practical level, I would suggest that it is this question of how to resist the *vigil* which makes the exploration of care profoundly interesting, and of relevance to all those involved in care: both providers and recipients. If care can be both discipline and *gift*, then in situations of care there is always the potential for that which is positive, enabling and empowering to become (intentionally or unintentionally, explicitly or without being noted) a possessive, controlling discourse. To give an example: in a therapeutic setting, a person undergoing treatment may well invest trust and confidence in a therapist, reciprocating an investment on the part of the therapist to enable the patient to take control of her or his situation. These investments may enable the patient to grow and break free of the constraints of suffering and dependency. But if these investments become codified – within discourses of professionalism, or as is sometimes the case in caring settings, within a repetition of a parent–child dependency (Parsons and Fox 1952, Forrester 1990, Fox 1993a) – then what was an empowering relationship becomes disempowerment. What might have enabled such growth becomes more to do with power and control: in Foucauldian terms, an inscription of identity and subjectivity.

3. It is intended that the explorations which follow will supply a more optimistic evaluation of care than that generally found in sociological writing. While sociology rightly re-evaluates discourses on care emanating from professional groups (and this chapter is part of that corpus), much of this critique has been concerned with dominance and control in care. Structuralist and Marxist analyses of health and welfare found a negative aspect to caring in the dominance arising from professional closure, patriarchy, capitalism or bureaucracy (Graham 1983, Lynch 1989, Stacey 1988, Ungerson 1987), or in 'unprofessional' labelling and stigmatization of patients (de Swaan 1990, Goffman 1970). Foucauldian analyses of discourses on care and welfare services (Armstrong 1983, Rose 1989, Nettleton 1992), and the studies which examine care in terms of 'emotional labour' (Hochschild 1983, James 1989) also contribute to a pessimism about the progressiveness of 'care'.

Such analyses of care do not do justice to the positive elements of care, nor to the investments by millions of carers – lay, voluntary and professional – who daily invest their efforts with love and generosity of spirit, such as the hospice care described in James (1989). Most people have at some time or other been the donor or the recipient of trust, unselfish generosity or love, and to argue that care can *only* be a technology of power (that is, the *vigil*) paints only part of the picture. The *vigil* of care is a technology of power, but the possibility of resisting that technology does not of itself entail a rejection of the caring which is given, but only a refusal to acquiesce in the subjectivity which the *vigil* of 'care' would produce in its subjects.

Finally, it will become clear that the transformation of the caring contact entailed in the promotion of this resistance is far-reaching, and fragments the present role of 'professional carer' irrevocably, replacing the carer/client relationship with one based not in dependency but in generosity and love. While this position is unlikely to be attractive to those in caring professions for whom the 'professionalism' associated with caring work is in itself a highly prized value, I would add that my argument is not anti-intellectual. Clearly it is important that the techniques of caring are subject to reflection, appraisal and quality control (Dolan 1993).

The Vigil: Care as Discipline

While care as an unselfish and loving giving of succour and support in response to others' suffering (care-as-gift) may be traced to Christian notions of love and charity, and was reflected in the early hospital establishments throughout the Christian world (Dolan 1993), social theorists have been quick to point to the less attractive aspects of the practice of care. Those discourses which held up the loving care of familial relationships as an example for care services have been criticized for ignoring the politics of the domestic setting (Graham 1979, Dunlop 1986). Meanwhile the genealogies of a range of health and welfare services demonstrate a discontinuous but endless fabrication of particular subjectivities in its 'clientele' (Armstrong 1983, Foucault 1976, 1979, Rose 1989).

In English, the word 'discipline' means both a set of practices by which individuals become subjects of power, and secondly a professional or academic grouping. The connection between these meanings has been illustrated in post-structuralist writing (Foucault 1976, 1979, 1988b, Goldstein 1984, Rose 1989), the common thread being the discourses by which knowledge both informs practice and supplies the authority for a group's claim to status and control. The association of power with knowledge suggests that in the context of care, the professionalization of caring (creating a discipline) cannot but lead to a disciplining of care's clients.

Recognizing this duality, Gardner (1992) argues that caring is paradoxical. On one hand, care is based upon relations which value giving, concern and enabling of the person who is cared for. On the other, the codification of caring practices and the formulation of a body of knowledge creates disciplines of caring which supply the basis for the authority and power of those who practise care, and in the process constructs the 'docile bodies' (Foucault 1979) of the recipients of care. Care is both an activity which meets some expressed need by another person, and the activity by which practitioners can claim that they are doing something called 'caring', and that this is appropriate, legitimate and valuable. Gardner suggests that the

> caring dimension of nursing helps to establish the independent practice area of nursing, and the growth in professionalism endows caring with a strength that did not exist when it was viewed as a 'weak' form of occupational behaviour. (1992: 251)

If this is the case, then the organization of care from Florence Nightingale to the present day is not only about caring *per se*, but also is the story of control and the fabrication of knowledge concerning 'care'.

This construction of a discipline of power/knowledge entails a technology of surveillance, and it is this regime which I call the *vigil* of care. To offer an explicit definition, the *vigil* is *the continual subjection of care's clients and increasingly, all aspects of the environment in which they live to the vigilant scrutiny of carers, and the consequent fabrication and perpetuation of subjectivities as 'carer' and 'cared-for'.*

By recourse to some recent care theory, I want to demonstrate how the *vigil* underpins care-as-discipline. Access to, and observation of, the carers' client group and the activities of caring are essential for the formulation of theory; just as access to and observation of patients was crucial for the development of medical discourse (Foucault 1976). But technical skills and practical experience are not in themselves sufficient to construct the crucial body of knowledge claimed by a profession. Clients must be researched and analysed, concludes Shrock, reflecting upon the professionalization of health visiting

> ... occupations aspiring to professional status therefore emphasise relevant and appropriate research activities, attempt to construct a

for their activities, identify concepts, principles and
.04)

rock continues, are questionable aims for a group whose
cilitation of self-knowledge among its clients. The down-
.onalization of care is captured beautifully in the following:

> When a candidate at interview is asked why she (sic) chose nursing the
> correct answer is no longer 'I want to help people'. If that is what she
> actually feels it would be more prudent to talk about social obligations,
> nursing being a profession which involved relating to others, career
> mobility, academic and emotional gratification. ... The value upon care
> remains high, but care is no longer 'tender' and 'loving', it is a specifi-
> able commodity ... A nurse no longer has a vocation; she has a
> profession. She is no longer dedicated; she is professional. She is no
> longer moral; she is accountable. (Inglesby 1992: 54)

The theorizing of care-as-profession can be traced in the discourses of
professionals and academics, and the continual devising of new 'models'
of care (for example, Bevis 1982, Brykczynska 1992, Kershaw 1992,
Lynaugh and Fagin 1988, Riehl and Roy 1980, Salvage 1989). An edited
collection entitled *Towards a Discipline of Nursing* (Gray and Pratt 1991)
documents the efforts to professionalize a caring group. This volume was
published to coincide with the translation of Australian pre-registration
nurse education from hospitals into a college setting. Gray and Pratt
outline their programme for the fabrication of a knowledge base for the
discipline: it must adopt science as its framework, to achieve the goals of
research, education and development of skills as scientific investigators as
well as clinical expertise (1991: 4–8).

Contributors to the collection variously discuss the contribution of
philosophical theory to the making of the discipline. Sims asserts the
importance of developing theory for successful nursing practice (1991:
51ff.); Anderson maps out an 'integrated health breakdown and intervention model' (1991: 108) fabricating its own concept of health as a
maximization of potential and expression in everyday activities of life
(ibid.: 109); while Cameron-Traub asserts the advantages for nursing
theory of a catholic approach, encompassing

> ... alternative conceptualisations of nursing as meeting patients' needs,
> interactive processes of the nurse–patient dyad, outcomes for the
> patient, or influences on human-environment patterning. (1991: 37)

Such positions construct – in ways which compare with the similar fabrications of the medical gaze – not only the caring profession itself, but also its clients, and it is in this sense that it seems appropriate to typify a *vigil* of care. Patient-centredness, while offering a contrast with medico-centric practices, is also effective in extending the gaze of the carer. Thomas and Dolan argue that

> The nurse where appropriate, must be able to follow the client and be sufficiently skilled and adaptable to care in any environment, be it the ward, day case unit or community. (1993: 125)

Later they suggest that this will mean that

> Nurses will play a more pro-active role in the maintenance of health and in providing primary, secondary and tertiary health education. Nurses of the 21st century will be actively involved in directing change and be adaptable to a changing world without fear of that change. (ibid.: 129)

For Clark (1993), the skills of the modern nurse encompass communication 'with all kinds of people in all kinds of setting', working in partnership with patients and informal carers, assessing environments, decision-making without recourse to colleagues and peers, and ensuring continuity of care. Twinn (1991) argues that the gaze of the health visitor is extensive, and includes not only individual advice-giving, but also counselling, profiling of communities' health and community development work.

The emphasis on surveillance within caring, and its association of knowledge and power, has been identified in studies of health visiting by Bloor and McIntosh (1990) and Mayall and Foster (1989). The latter authors suggest that within a framework of the profession's concern with child health surveillance, visits to families which from a health visitor's perspective is 'dropping in' or 'popping in', from a parental viewpoint is 'inspection of child-care standards'. Miles (1988) found that health visitors and social workers caused mothers anxiety that they would be defined as 'non-coping', resulting in their children being taken into care.

The point which I am making by reference to these theories of care-as-profession is that, although there are good and principled reasons for generating such discourses, unintentionally but necessarily, the construction of disciplines of care affects those who are cared for. The centrality of the cared-for as the subjects which give caring disciplines their authority, cannot help but construct them within particular subjectivities. At the most basic level, caring professionals' establishment of a divide between themselves and those for whom they care – labelling them as clients or patients (Hugman 1991: 113ff.) – creates a subjectivity for the cared-for which is then to be played out in the gaze of the *vigil*.

Further, there seems to be a momentum to the theorization of care, in which the subject of care becomes substrate rather than focus. In the Gray and Pratt collection mentioned above, and a volume edited by Dolan (1993) to celebrate and reflect upon the UK Project 2000 (which similarly shifts nurse education into an academic setting), the patient remains the focus: her or his presence moderating the extent to which she or he is fabricated. But in a North American text on the nursing profession, the patient is little more than a spectre. Strumpf and Stevenson's assessment of the knowledge and skills required for advanced gerontologic nursing by a nursing specialist 'holding, at a minimum, a master's degree in geronto-logic nursing' (1992: 422) includes not only understanding of pathological and psychosocial factors in ageing, but the skills to

- Employ clinical reasoning
- Provide comprehensive nursing services independently or as part of a team
- Develop, offer and evaluate services
- Work with professionals and clients to explore and resolve ethical problems
- Provide consultation and education to other professionals
- Provide leadership and advocacy for elderly clients
- Collaborate, use and disseminate research
- Provide professional leadership
- Participate in continuing education, certification and evaluation of standards of nursing practice. (ibid)

This contribution is drawn from Aiken and Fagin's (1992) *Agenda for the 1990s,* a volume which ranges widely to cover professional and policy issues in nursing, financing of care, specialization and education. In the same way that medical texts have imprinted their objects of study as collections of tissues, cells or chemical processes, Aiken and Fagin have decentred the carer/cared-for contact. They build an edifice of theory and professional discourse which no longer refers explicitly to the business of nursing patients, although the absent subject of care is ultimately the resource which sustains the authority of the discourse.

In summary, the construction and strengthening of disciplinary markers of knowledge shift the balance of power away from clients and patients towards health professionals, as discourses such as those outlined here identify and achieve distinctive perspectives on 'care-as-discipline'. However, I do not wish to leave the analysis here. Certainly, analyses of care and caring which uncritically identify it as an unquestionably 'good thing' get it wrong. But so do readings which implicate caring as a disciplinary procedure pure and simple. Caring has a dual character: on one hand, it has the potential to subject the cared-for within discourses of power/knowledge (the *vigil*). On the other, and differently constituted, it can supply the possibility of resistance to discourse on the part of the person who is in need of care. How to achieve the latter in place of the former is the subject of the next section.

Resisting the Vigil: Care-as-Gift

The *vigil* of care is the disciplinary technology which, through professionalism and theory, fabricates and inscribes those who are cared for. It reminds us of the vigilance which Florence Nightingale emphasized in her programme for the nursing profession, and the subsequent technologies which enabled her successors to mount their vigil over their patients and clients. In the previous chapter I looked at spatial organization as a technology of control: the Nightingale ward with its central nursing station provided the basis for her philosophy of surveillance. Modern technologies of observation now enable flexibility in hospital design, but the principle remains. In the context of community-based care, the *vigil* is both to do with practice and with theory. It is reflected in the discourses (such as those documented earlier) of groups including health visitors, district nurses, social workers and other carers, including lay and voluntary carers, whose work takes them far beyond the gaze of the clinic (Foucault 1976) or the dispensary (Armstrong 1983), into their clients' homes and private lives.

It will already be clear that I have counterposed two concepts throughout this chapter, firstly 'care-as-discipline', and secondly 'care-as-gift'. In using the second I have anticipated the work upon which I will now draw, that of Derrida (1993, 1995) and the feminist post-structuralist Cixous, who has theorized two realms, those of the 'Gift' and the 'Proper' (Cixous 1986). Cixous's position is partly rooted in the analyses of Derrida (1976, 1978), whose considerations of undecidability and *différance* in language supplies the basis for resistance to discourse (Moi 1985). *Différance* is the inevitable displacement of any absolute reference point for a word, phrase or proposition: although words claim to refer to underlying realities, all they can ever refer to are other words and concepts. Because of this *undecidability* concerning meaning, no proposition can claim absolutely to represent the world; there is always the possibility of other interpretations, and which interpretation is accepted is more to do with power than with accuracy or truthfulness.

Cixous (1986) opposes *gift* relationships (which she sees as feminine) with the masculine realm of the *proper*: of property, propriety, possession, identity and dominance. The characteristics of *gift* relationships would seem particularly apposite for relations entailing care, and might include such features of engagement as generosity, trust, confidence, love, benevolence, commitment, delight, patience, esteem, admiration and curiosity.

But these relations quickly slip into other more possessive constructs: trust becomes dependency, esteem becomes reverence, generosity becomes patronage, curiosity becomes the *vigil*. We might also note how few of these words are part of the discourse of professional care, indeed, which suggests relations which could be seen as *unprofessional* and inappropriate to the highly theorized, formalized care documented in textbooks, in which the carer/cared-for distinction is so strong and so impenetrable (Fox 1993a). Care in the realm of the *proper* is a possessive controlling relationship which constantly requires its subject to behave in certain ways, to be defined as 'patient' or 'client', and to repeat the patterns of those who have been the objects of 'care' before.

The force and value of this distinction between the *gift* and the *proper* rests in the possibility that things could be different. It offers the potential for an ethics and politics of engagement based on a celebration of difference, not of identity (Haber 1994). The *proper* is a possessive relationship, constantly requiring of its object that it behaves in certain ways, that it is defined (as 'patient', 'nurse', 'carer'), and repeats the patterns of those who have been the objects of its discourse previously. Substituting *gift* relationships changes everything: we engage with others now as others, not as those with whom we might wish to identify. Definition is replaced with metaphor and allusion, analysis and theory with poetics and expression, professional care by love and the celebration of difference.

The notion of the gift is not new in sociology. The Durkheimian sociologist Mauss (1990) wrote a classic monograph in the 1920s on the role of the gift in various societies, and the significance of a gift as a form of social bonding based in obligation and reciprocity has been addressed by Hochschild (1983: 80–2). But let me be clear what I mean when I speak of a *gift*, because it is possible to have *proper* gifts! What Mauss and Hochschild describe in talking of 'gift economies' based in reciprocity are *proper* relationships, and in the realm of the *proper*, a gift is threatening because it establishes an inequality, a difference, an imbalance in power.

The act of giving becomes an act of aggression, an exposure of the Other (Moi 1985: 112). Caring services may disguise the exchange relationship by insurance or taxation schemes, but carer/cared-for relationships in the public realm retain such expectations. This expectation may be managed through compliance and docility on the parts of patients, or by a 'gratefulness' for the expertise of the carer. But if patients come to see that their efforts at reciprocity – to return something of what they are given – are inadequate, they are humiliated, degraded or stigmatized. They may try to offset their dependency with demands, complaints and accusation (de Swaan 1990: 36, also see Hochschild 1983: 80–2 for a discussion of reciprocity in emotional giving).

Gifts may serve many different purposes. In recent work on the care offered by volunteers, I found that voluntary caring was rarely undertaken for altruistic reasons, but for reasons of career progression, brushing up skills, or simply to get out of the house and do something to fill the day. These volunteers gained much from their interactions with those for whom they cared, often to the point where one wondered what the recipient got back! In contrast, the *gift* is not given with any expectation of reciprocity; in the realm of the gift, those who give do not expect gratefulness or even an acknowledgement of their effort. The true *gift* is one which one does not even realize one is giving (Derrida 1992).

Thinking about the politics of this latter kind of *gift* relationship suggests that it is less to do with the kinds of 'negative' resistance by the subjects of care documented by Bloor and McIntosh (1990) in their study of health visitors' clients (for example, challenges to regulations, non-compliance and concealment), than with the Idea of a positive enabling investment. 'Care' has the capacity, within this formulation, either to be the discursive fabrication of a subjectivity upon the person who is cared for, or to be a *gift*. Such a *gift*, through its investment of generosity, enables a resistance to power/knowledge, supplying the cared-for person with a resource with which to challenge her or his subjectivity. Care-as-gift substitutes generosity with the *vigil*.

The two contrasting senses of care, 'care-as-discipline' grounded in the *proper* and constituted in the technology of the *vigil* and 'care-as-*gift*', an enabling generosity invested freely and without expectation, may reflect a historical move from the latter to the former aspect. Dunlop (1986) has suggested that the creation of an impersonal health-care system in the modern era supplied the basis for a discourse on 'care' and consequently a distinctive profession of nursing. These 'proper' elements of caring expertise and 'professionalism' are particular forms of power/knowledge, which fabricate the subjectivity of the cared-for. A relationship of generosity is replaced with a relationship of possession. If this is the case, then what does a 're-enchantment' of care, substituting the *proper* with the *gift*, mean?

A New Ethics and Politics of Care

The substitution of the *proper* with the *gift* in caring relationships supplies the possibility of a new ethics and politics in health care. If this is easy to say, then it seems that it is far harder in practice. Exploring care and the relationships between carers and those who receive care, I have been struck by the extent to which *proper* relations impinge on an area which – intuitively – one might expect to reflect the *gift*. We can see the ease with which a gift relationship becomes one of possession and repetition in Bond's study of the rationalization and formalizing of informal caring by family or friends as part of 'care in the community'. UK legislation provides the possibility of financially rewarding informal carers, and providing training to ensure standards of care are achieved. Bond argues that this professionalization of informal care leads to a loss of the 'caring-about' element of the relationship through four processes: the implementation of expert knowledge, the legitimation of care through medical judgements of health and illness, the individualization of behaviour and its consequent depoliticization (1991: 11–12). We see the substitution of the *vigil* for the *gift*, replacing the investments of love, admiration, commitment, accord, involvement, generosity which carers supply in caring with a relation of possession, in which the recipient of care is the property of the carer, upon whom the carer 'does' care. In place of the trust, confidence and esteem on the part of the recipient of care towards the carer are investments which make care synonymous with the relationship; the recipient of care enters into a relation of negative dependency.

While rationalization may be a response to material social relations, it can also be a response to the ontological threat of the caring relationship. To be in need of care can challenge many psychological and emotional aspects of our sense-of-self at the deepest level, as can the requirement to provide care to another. De Swaan's study of a cancer ward suggests the difficulties of contemplating a caring relationship based in generosity. Here, as de Swaan describes it, is a libidinal economy in which – while the anger and fear of patients may be distressingly manifest – the anxieties of staff caring for people who are dying are displaced or translated into medical terms. Patients' bodies are cared for, while their emotions go untended; staff do not discuss their upset with colleagues. Doctors and nurses learn not to become attached to seriously ill and dying people: the investment of care, affection and generosity by a member of staff in a patient goes 'unrewarded' when the next day the patient is dead (de Swaan 1990: 42–7). Yet sometimes, even at the level of physical caring, there are possibilities for a *gift*, enabling patients to 'become'.

> To patients it means much when doctors and nurses know how to handle their wounds competently and without fear. The nurse patiently washing a dilapidated patient, changing his clothes, is also the only one who dares touch him without disgust or fear, who quietly and compe- tently handles the body which so torments and frightens the patient … (who) knows how to deal skilfully with the wounds and lumps, in doing so liberating the patients for the moment from their isolation. (ibid.: 48)

This extract suggests how one is to understand the force of the *gift*: it is constituted in an open-endedness. It stands in place of theory, even a theory of liberation or empowerment (for example, Malin and Teasdale 1991). Such theory *tells* the other *how* to be more free or more sexy or more something else, closing down possibilities, making the other an appendage of the discourse, inscribed with the power of the Word. It does not say what something is, or is not: it allows, for a moment at least, a thing to become multiple, to be both something and another thing and another. Bunting offers as an example of such opening-up:

> … a family working with a child with special health needs. As the family members work with the child and with one another, each moves beyond the self and the present reality to the possibles that unfold … The family's health is the movement toward and the expression of these possibles as they are chosen and lived. (Bunting 1993: 14)

This notion of co-presence was a fundamental in Rosemarie Parse's devel- opment of a theory of 'health as human becoming' (Parse *et al.* 1985, Parse 1987). In Parse's view, such a becoming is

> the process of reaching beyond self towards the not-yet … The possibles arise from the multi-dimensional experiences and the context of situa- tions, and are opportunities from which alternatives are chosen. (1985: 12)

Collaboration and sharing is something which is picked up in Brykczynska when she suggests that

True caring involves growth, mutual growth of carer and cared-for; and it is this ability to grow, to change, to progress from pain to disintegration to purpose and equilibrium that gives the caring phenomena [sic] its impetus and rationale. (Brykczynska 1992: 237)

Yet even here it is necessary to ask what constitutes purpose and equilibrium, and by whom are these defined? There is no guarantee that acting in the world – through one's gifts of love, generosity and trust – will lead to another's becoming, even within such a perspective. Sometimes one's attempts to give (however well intended) do not enable but disable (Hochschild 1983: 81). Indeed the absence of any absolute 'true' reading of one's actions or words ensures that sometimes this will be so. Conversely, things we do may turn out, unintentionally, to be the most powerful gifts we can give.

Gifts and the Vigil: the Experience of Care

To understand more about how the *vigil* and the gift of care work, I undertook research on this topic in 1997. I wanted to find out about the experiences of people who were the recipients of care, and so I talked with older adults living in residential accommodation in Australia. It was obvious that these older people could identify the two poles of care without any prompting from me. First, the aspect of care which derives from a professional discipline and theory: the *vigil*. Echoing classic tales of the routinization of hospital life (Davis and Horobin 1977), some residents felt that they had to fit into the routines of the staff, or the organizational structures and processes.

> *Mr M:* I think the older staff are a bit more caring than the younger staff. The younger staff probably think, 'Oh, come on. Let's get going.' You know what it's like when you're young. You want to get moving and all that sort of stuff. You've only got a certain amount of time that they have to do things. And if this old bloke's holding them up, well, they get a bit agitated. They've got a routine to do every day, you see, and if they can't get on with their routine, well ...

> *Mr L:* There's a lot of other people in here. There's no continuity of the same girls coming to see you. Plus they're having agency girls in so you don't get to know people. Most people in here would like the same girls to come in.

Mrs L: Shower you, or to take you to the toilet. I've had everybody here take me to the toilet. It's a bit embarrassing you know, but I can't go on my own.

The disciplinary nature of the institution was reflected in the rules which were laid down. While these might often be formulated in the perceived best interests of the residents, they were sometimes seen as constraining.

Mrs S: I would love to get my hands on a couple of kilos of potatoes and peel them, do you understand? That I miss. It can't be done and you accept that. If ever the chance comes up, I would certainly take it. But I don't think there's any likelihood of it because, as I said, everything is prepared when it comes in. I think it's a pity that we don't. We have got the facilities here that we could prepare some ... and I would be perfectly willing to be in that.
What do you think you would get from doing that? Would it be to use your skills ...?
Mrs S: A little bit of satisfaction perhaps. I haven't done any cooking for a couple of years now. Perhaps to be able to say 'Well, I cooked that', you know.

Mrs Y: I've got some steps in that cupboard that I can put up and stand on for them but there's always the chance that you could fall. They'd be very cross with me if they came in and found me on the floor. You just have to be careful, but you don't have to watch television if you don't want to. And I don't. I think people think I'm a bit peculiar. Probably I am.

Even when the rules did not immediately affect a resident, the existence of the regime of care – with its regulations and routines – was a source of upset or fear.

Mrs Y: No, well I may not like it either when I have to have someone coming in when I have a shower. I can have my shower now on my own and I have my shower in the morning but my neighbour has to have her shower at night and she can only have a shower every other night. I won't like it when I have to do that because I'm used to having my shower when I'm ready. I won't like it if I can only have a shower every other day. I won't like that at all.

More generally, a loss of sense of autonomy and responsibility for oneself could be experienced as restricting and disheartening.

Mrs A: The worst thing about it really is, I think, you lose your responsibility when you come into these sort of places and you haven't got that, you know, to be responsible for – the shopping, the cleaning, the cooking and everything. And when you come in here, or any of these places, you haven't got that responsibility and it's not good to have no responsibility for anything. And that is very hard.

In some circumstances, the disciplinary nature of the care setting took on an oppressive character, with one resident voicing anxiety about the consequences of resisting.

Mr L: Some girls are very good, very caring, some others it's just a day's work to them. Each person has got a care list but in a lot of cases the girls don't even read it. They don't know what they're supposed to do. They say they haven't got time to read it and we have had the Ageing Rights Advocacy here and it's in their statement that the girls should read everybody's nursing care plan so that they know what they've got to do. But if you upset the girls, they can make it awkward for you.

These negative comments about being cared for in an institutional setting were counter-balanced by a clear perception by many residents of positive aspects to the care they received.

Mrs A: The people are special. They're always bright and cheerful and willing to help as much as they can. And the people like down in reception, people in charge of sections and that, they are all special sort of people. You have to be if you're looking after old people in all sorts of conditions wouldn't you?
What do you think it takes for somebody to be that special kind of person?
Mrs A: I think they'd have to be generous and I do think they're special because they're patient with the residents.
Mr A: They put up with a lot.

Mrs G: Well, they have got to have a lot of patience I think. Because we can get a bit cantankerous in our old age. But I think these are very nice people. Very, very nice. They are hard-working girls too. I love them to death.

Asked what made a good carer, the residents offered a range of comments which reflect the notion of the *gift* developed earlier in this chapter.

Mr O: A genuine interest in your welfare. Yes. I think it's the old cliché 'Do unto others as you would have done unto you.' I can't go further than that. It's simply that.

Mrs S: I think it's an understanding of people. I think if you can judge a person, you know what they want. I'm pretty sure that's what it is. I think back to myself, 'Now would I like that?' or 'Would I like somebody to do that for me?' and sort of take it from there. I wouldn't like to be treated like, 'I don't care' and I wouldn't do that to anybody else.

Mrs St: Well, love is just so different than caring for a person – it's compassion. I could care for you and say 'Come on and do this', rather than gently putting my arm around you and saying 'Just come on and we'll do so and so.' But love is just giving and giving of yourself and there's certainly different kinds of love.
What is it like to receive that love, when you are on the other end, when you are being cared for?
Mrs St: Well I see it like comfort and it also gives you confidence and security. Especially if you are feeling sort of down and someone shows you just that extra bit of care or love or whatever. It certainly makes you feel a lot better than somebody breezing in and saying 'Now listen here. Just come on and we'll do this.' It's the tone of voice.
So it makes you feel good about yourself?
Mrs St: Yes I think so. If you are giving and helping a person or helping somebody else in some way, surely you yourself don't think you are a great person, but it gives you some sort of satisfaction, doesn't it? If you do something kind or help somebody, you give out that you are a caring person.

If residents found aspects of their care which were positive, while recognizing other attributes as negative, this did not mean that they were passive in the face of the constraints. One couple in the hostel accommodation had faced the routines and transformed a routine of care into a gift.

Mr L: When we first came here they didn't do Joyce's hair or her make-up and I went down to the head office and I said to the manager, 'You like to have your hair done and your make-up on, don't you?' 'Oh, yes' she said. 'Well that's how Joyce likes to feel in the morning.' I said, 'If a person thinks they look good, they feel good.' So they started doing her hair.

And for some residents, the care they received, even if it did reflect a dependency, was not perceived as constraint, but as a freedom or liberation.

> *Mrs H:* On the whole I think it's lovely here. What could you wish for anything better than this? I am, I feel independent. I don't ask anybody to do anything that I can't do myself. And the nurses come here and help me with my shower. They don't shower me altogether. They just help me with different things I can't reach or anything. You see I can't stand once I get into the shower because I've only got one leg. And if I let go, I'm gone. So they're always there to help me up and down off the seat and that.

These extracts support the dichotomous character of care which has been developed in this chapter. On one hand, the care which these older adults receive is codified and organized in rules, routines and plans: the *vigil*. On the other, it is experienced as fulfilling and liberating. The epithets of generosity, patience and love are ascribed both to the care and the carers: precisely the terms which constitute the *gift* of care as set out earlier. This data suggests that, at least in institutional settings, the *vigil* and the *gift* go hand in hand. However much a regime of care aims to be supportive and empowering to its subjects, it will be perceived by some as constraining and oppressive.

In the context of this book's theme of going *beyond health*, I want to argue at this point that we can see in this opposition the conflict between power and control on one hand, and – on the other – the resistance to that power. But what is important is to recognize that resistance is not necessarily a solitary response to control. We may find allies in unexpected places, gifts which the givers do not even realize they are giving. For these older adults, the carers may be important allies in their struggle to maximize their potential. Conversely, the valiant and well-meaning efforts by people to help, empower or give to others may not be perceived as any of these things, but as a further codification of life: contributing to an act of power. Unfortunately there may be no way of assuring the former and avoiding the latter. In the final section of this chapter I want to reflect on the consequences of this analysis for the professions and others who are involved in caring.

Beyond Professionalism?

I suggested earlier that care was paradoxical, and I have outlined the conflicts between the two irreconcilable elements of care, as *vigil* and as *gift*. I would suggest that this paradox has faced carers as they have sought to valorize their activities. I can illustrate this by reference to James's writing on emotional labour in a hospice. Emotional labour, she found, was an important contribution to a 'guiding ideology' of 'total care', defined as

> the social, spiritual, emotional and physical care [which] encompasses elements of care which are usually obscured in medical settings ... and require management and attention in the same way that physical symptoms do. (1989: 20)

In James's study, staff saw emotional labour as integral to their jobs, but something which tended to get a low priority in comparison with pressing demands for physical care (ibid.: 32–5). Emphasizing the importance of this emotional work, James is part of a movement in nursing to find a new conception of 'total' or 'holistic' care to underpin nursing theory, and in turn to enhance the status of nursing as a profession. Yet I argued earlier in the chapter that such moves to professionalize care could turn something with the potential to be empowering into something controlling. In this way, a *gift* of care becomes codified and turns into a further element of the disciplinary *vigil* of care.

To address this paradox for the professions based in care (and perhaps health professions more generally), it is helpful to reflect on these conflicting relations in terms of ethical engagement with others. Modernism and humanism have, in their pursuit of rationality, relativized moral codes (Bauman 1989, Caputo 1993), yet White argues (1991) that the underlying and unacknowledged ethic of modernism is a *will to mastery*. This can be seen in the emphasis in modern medicine upon the heroic, where the attempt to succeed has sometimes come to be held in greater esteem than any possible benefits of action (Fox 1994, Knowles 1977). At the root of any such claim to justify intervention is the *responsibility to act* (White 1991); theories and codes of professional conduct underpin such active engagement – potentially regardless of outcome or impact. Along with other postmodern writers (Bauman 1993b, Haber 1994), White goes on to connect postmodern concerns with *difference* with an ethics based in a *responsibility to otherness*. The latter is the rejection of a will to mastery, and the substitution of this *proper*, identity-seeking discourse with a *gift* relation, in which that which is other, different and diverse is celebrated. White suggests that the 'mood' of such an engagement based in a *gift* might be one of 'grieving delight'. Quietly allowing the recognition of mortality and limitations of human affairs into everyday life, this mood would come alive in the spacing between the self and otherness. The delight with the appearance of the other brings with it the urge to draw it closer. But that urge must realise its limits, beyond which the drawing nearer becomes a gesture of grasping. And that realisation will be palpable only when we are sensitive to the appearance of the particular other as testimony of finitude. Then delight will be paired with a sense of grief or mourning at the fragility and momentary quality of the appearance of the other. (1991: 90)

Grief sensitizes us to injustice, while the element of delight deepens the concern with fostering difference: love and difference.

An ethos of a responsibility to otherness requires a radically different conception of human potential or its failing, and of what constitutes the 'care' which engages with this potential. The objective of care in this perspective is to do with becoming and possibilities, about resistance to discourse, and a generosity towards otherness. It is a process which offers promise, rather than fulfilling it, offers possibility in place of certainty, multiplicity in place of repetition, difference in place of identity. It is the *gift* which expects no recognition.

Having argued earlier in this chapter that theorizing care generates a disciplinary *vigil*, it is clearly absurd to try to theorize (in the sense of laying down a formula or generality) how to be free of the *vigil*. So, if we are to have a 'manifesto' of the *gift*, it may have to be limiting, rather than all-encompassing (a 'grand' narrative). It might go something like this:

- If you have to take sides, be on the side of the nomad thought: the wandering nomad broken free (for however short a time) from a territory (see chapter 5 for more on nomads and territories). From such a position comes the reflection that acting is to be judged in terms of its consequences, not by any overarching discourse of good or truth.
- If you must have values, celebrate difference and otherness. Structures and systems force us into sameness. Recognize the undecidability and openness of the world, its capacity always to become other.
- If you must desire anything, desire in a spirit of generosity, not for mastery. Do not try to possess the object of your desire (the *other*); make it possible that your relationship is a gift requiring no response or repetition. Accept the gifts which others may make available to you, and take pleasure in them for their own sake.

Love and difference. The promise of postmodernism for the engagements which we call 'caring' concerns the reintroduction of the emotional, the non-rationalistic into those interactions. To use Bauman's (1993a) term, it is a *re-enchantment* following the disenchantment of modernity with its emphasis on the secular and the rational. Needless to say, this cuts against the grain of modernist disciplines which have based their authority on the knowledge generated by their *gaze* and their *vigil*. Basing care in a relationship of a *gift* necessarily evens out the power relations between client and practitioner, teacher and student, all such engagements become (to subvert Tuckett *et al.*'s (1985) phrase) *meetings between novices*. It forces us to reflect upon what it is to be human, and to engage with other human beings. Care grounded in an ethics and politics of love and difference means there is no longer a simple recipe for a caring which enables; no formula can provide the answer. Just as a celebration of difference entails an abandonment of tried and tested formulae, any such formula would offer nothing other than a new discourse on 'how to do caring'. But we can point to the kinds of activities within caring which constitute the *vigil*, and reflect that there is always the possibility of resistance, that anything we do is potentially a *gift*, that things can be different, and take it from there.

Part 2
RESISTANCE

Introduction

Modernism – the way of thinking about the world which privileges science and reason, and self-consciously ruptures from the past (Wood *et al.* 1998: 1734) – has provided us with much of what has become the landscape and architecture of the academic disciplines of science and social science. Released from the established view in the medieval period that the world might be known only with God's help, modernist thinking argued that if only the problem could be adequately enunciated, and the methods for observing a phenomenon appropriately worked out and applied, then that phenomenon would yield up its secrets. Knowledge of the world would be simply a matter of incrementalism, as the questions were formulated and the methods found to seek answers.

It was inevitable that this enterprise of chasing truth through observation and theory-building and testing would turn its sights on human beings themselves. In this reflexive moment, as Foucault has suggested (1970), were the social sciences born, and since that date, the dissecting of humanity has become the property of psychology, sociology and anthropology and political science. Philosophy, ethics and theology have been relegated to the sidelines in the face of this onslaught from those who believe truth can come from observation and the theorizing built on such observation.

Given the underpinning cosmology of modernism, with the human mind at the centre, and human reason as the means of discovering all there is to know, it is hardly surprising that this view of the world has privileged a human self which is free, prior and (more or less) independent of its environment. The pre-modern soul has been replaced with a self which is equally *essential*.

Essentialism has many guises. It can be seen in the romantic conception of the human subject buffeted by the forces of history, but capable of transcending these vicissitudes: triumphing or in defeat becoming an icon of all that makes us human. Romanticism's privileging of the human subject is a reflection of its humanistic roots, and in parallel, humanistic movements in psychology and sociology are also grounded in this essentialist approach to the self. We can see this most clearly in those humanistic forms of sociology such as interactionism and phenomenology. Both these perspectives emphasize agency, and argue that the social world is a constructed consequence of the sense-making activities of individuals (for example, see the work of Shutz (1962) and Berger and Luckmann (1971) on the social construction of reality).

A range of theories which deal with socialization also involve a notion of an essential self. The idea that 'the child is father of the man' is fundamental to developmental psychology (for instance, in the work of Piaget and Erickson). In these theories, the self is present, albeit in an unformed state, from birth. The period of childhood is not only one of bodily growth, but also of maturation of the self through the processes of primary and secondary socialization. Even in perspectives which emphasize structure, such as the theories of Marx and Weber, there is an implicit if not explicit essentialism of self. Thus for Marx, the oppressive and unfair forces of capitalism are to be shed like chains: for Weber, capitalism and industrialization created an 'iron cage' of bureaucracy which constrained the individual.

However, a number of perspectives have challenged this essentialism of self. We can see this in part in Goffman's work, in which he applies a dramaturgical model of the social: individuals live out their lives wearing a series of masks. Similarly, in ethnomethodology there is a sense that our social lives are committed to perfecting a range of roles, so we can 'do being human'. In neither of these perspectives is it entirely clear whether there is anything of substance behind the mask, or whether – like Peer Gynt – when we strip away the layers that make up the self like the integuments of an onion, we find there is nothing left in the centre. In anthropological structuralism, the emphasis upon structure is complete, and there is little room for any sense of an agentic self. Ritual and myth structure the ways in which humans see and understand the world around them, with culture as the outcome.

These structuralist approaches have been seen as the avatars of post-structuralism, which most explicitly reject an essentialism of self. Thus in the work of Foucault, the self is nothing more than an epiphenomenon of the systems of thought or 'discourses' which structure subjectivity. Unlike the earlier structuralists, here subjectivity and self are outcomes of the *micropolitics* of power, rather than gross social structures.

An anti-essentialist model of the self has the advantage that it does not require a theory of subjectivity as prior and foundational to the human being. Rather the self is a consequence of the impact of forces of the social, thus explaining the socialization of individuals into their own cultures. On the other hand, an anti-essentialist approach to subjectivity is problematic for a number of reasons. First, it is counter-factual to lived experience: we do have a sense of the continuity of our selves, and of being, at least in part, free from the constraints of the world in which we live. Second, and concomitantly, it is clear that the forces of the social, whether conceptualized as macro-structures, or a micropolitics, are not in themselves sufficient to explain either the patterning of human history or the everyday variation in human activities. Human beings do have the capacity to resist, and also a disconcerting tendency to interpret the same social situation in a variety of ways.

For these reasons, an anti-essentialist model of self has to address issues of agency and resistance. In this section of the book, I endeavour to set out such a model. This model will provide the basis for a theory of a resisting subject capable of moving *beyond health*. Chapter 4 devotes considerable space to an analysis of power and resistance in the work of Michel Foucault. Foucault has been extremely influential in post-structuralist thought over the past two decades, but I would argue that because of the approach he developed – his position is deficient as the basis for a theory of resistance. For these reasons, in chapter 5, I move to the work of Deleuze and Guattari to explore the anti-essentialist model of self which they call the *Body-without-Organs*. Deleuze and Guattari provide the basis for a theory of *nomadology* or subjectivity free from the constraints of the social.

Ultimately the choice between essentialist and anti-essentialist models of self cannot be made on the basis of the available evidence. We simply do not have the data that would enable us to decide between these alternatives. Essentialist models have traditionally been favoured by those committed to a project of emancipation or liberation, and with those on the progressive wing of politics. Denying any absolute sense of right or justice, post-structuralists such as Lyotard and Baudrillard have been labelled as conservative or reactionary. This I believe misses the point. While an anti-essentialist model of the self strips away any foundationalist notion of 'human rights' or the possibility of a Habermasian community based on shared understanding, it opens the way for a new *politics of difference* which favours diversity over identity, becoming over being. The political and ethical commitment of an anti-essentialism of self will be fully developed in the final section of the book.

4
Beyond Foucault's Docile Body

In the first section of this book, we considered the impact of power on humans, their bodies and how they think of themselves. Throughout those chapters, we acknowledged how people's lives were constrained by acts of power: In Lyotard's vocabulary, how power framed what could be experienced, what could be spoken, and what must remain silent. Power is thus a feature of embodiment and subjectivity, and if we wish to move *beyond* health, we need to understand power. A constant theme in those chapters, and one with which this second section of the book is concerned, is with resistance to that power.

Moving beyond health is not theoretical activity. However, if we are to understand resistance, we need the right theoretical tools. Because the work of Michel Foucault has offered us a sophisticated analysis of power, it could be argued that it is to this body of work which we should turn. In this chapter I want to argue that this is mistaken. Foucault's position does not offer us a satisfactory model for resistance to power. Because this position is so influential, I shall devote considerable space to an analysis of Foucault's theory, to demonstrate why I am unhappy with his model. Then, in the next chapter, I shall consider an alternative reading deriving from the work of Deleuze and Guattari (1988).

Foucault, of course, was a philosopher. However, his work has become influential in a range of disciplines, including sociology and cultural studies. Within sociology, Foucault's writing has supplied a different understanding of power from analyses deriving from Weberian and Marxist theory (Nettleton 1995: 8–13 *passim*). His 'empirical' analyses of historical and archival materials have been taken up with enthusiasm within sub-disciplinary groupings in sociology, notably health and illness, sociologies of gender and the body, social welfare and organizational sociology. In these fields, Foucauldian approaches have been applied to offer a critique of many features of modernity and the modern subject. Indeed, it has been claimed (Silverman 1985, Eckermann 1997: 155) that Foucault's perspective successfully bridges the agency/structure dichotomy which has been such an issue within sociology.

However, closer examination of this 'sociological Foucault' (Goldstein 1984) suggests the complexities of the decentring of self and the 'deep structure' conception of the rules of discursive formation may not have been fully addressed. In this chapter, my argument will be that Foucault's ontology is itself ambiguous and contradictory, and this ambiguity may be carried over into Foucauldian sociology. Such ambiguity is not necessarily a fatal flaw (perhaps indeed it is an antidote to modernist meta-narrative), nor need we be 'faithful' to Foucault (Armstrong 1997: 15). However, I would argue that sociologists who wish to apply the approach should critically appraise the implications of Foucault's ontology, and remain extremely cautious when extrapolating (and perhaps subtly adapting) the position to meet sociological ends.

Foucault was critical of theories which consider power as 'sovereign': a unitary and centralized construct (Foucault 1980b: 115, Wickham, 1986: 169) and hence primarily repressive in character. A principal technology of power, Foucault argued (1976, 1979, 1980a), is the *gaze*, which is concerned with the gathering of information, to inform and create a discourse on its subject-matter. Discourses create *effects of truth* which are of themselves neither true nor false (Foucault 1980b: 116–19). Because of this association of a productive power with the fabrication of effects of truth, Foucault speaks of *power/knowledge* – a phenomenon which cannot be reduced simply to either component. Armstrong (1983) succinctly sums up this association:

> Power assumes a relationship based on some knowledge which creates and sustains it; conversely, power establishes a particular regime of truth in which certain knowledges become admissible or possible. (1983: 10)

A range of studies in sociology has used a Foucauldian model to document these knowledges or 'knowledgeabilities'. For example, patriarchy (Sawicki 1991, Weedon 1987), masculinity (Hearn and Morgan 1990), architecture (Prior 1988), criminology (Pfohl and Gordon 1988), community medicine and public health (Armstrong 1983, 1994, Lupton 1995, Petersen 1997), dentistry (Nettleton 1992), developmental psychology (Rose 1989, Tyler 1997), religion (Moore 1994, Paden 1988), pornography (Kaite 1988), education (Goodson and Dowbiggin 1990, Grant 1997), beauty and fitness (Glassner 1989, Probyn 1988), and death (Prior 1987). In many of these studies, the gaze of power, operating through modernist techniques of surveillance, supplies the raw material for a discourse which turns people into subjects of professions (or disciplines). The power and authority of such disciplines are played out in the everyday encounters between professionals (or privileged others) and their subject-matter, be they children, patients or clients, workers, family members or lovers. In other words, power/knowledge is implicated in the formation of subjectivity.

This relation between power and subjectivity is clearly of interest to social and cultural theorists, and the attraction of Foucault's formulation may be related to its apparent transcendence of both structuralism and humanism (Dreyfus and Rabinow 1982, Smart 1985: 16). It breaks with structuralism in that it denies that power is something which is merely coercive in a traditional Marxist or Weberian perspective (Pizzorno 1992). It marks a break with humanism inasmuch as it decentres the individual as the prior agent in creating the social world, rejecting subjectivity as something essential, prior to discourse, which power acts against. Power is a productive process, creating human subjects and their capacity to act (Butler 1990: 139). Even what are apparently self-empowering practices (such as liberation from sexual prohibitions, or 'self-actualization') are the workings of new reflexive technologies of power (Foucault 1984, 1985).

But how useful is this model for the study of identity and embodiment, and for our project of embodiment beyond health? Foucault was himself able to develop philosophical and quasi-historical analyses, but his position rendered him relatively politically impotent (Ostrander 1988: 180). The reasons for such impotence and the kinds of manipulation/glossing/silencing of Foucault's positions which are made by sociologists to meet the objectives of an engaged (and embodied) sociology, will be explored more fully in the next three sections, which consider the ontological status of discourse, body and self in his work.

The Foucauldian Ontology of Discourse

The centrality of the concept of discourse in Foucault's work, and its association with knowledge and power, suggest a continuity between his project and the sociology of knowledge; in particular the kinds of approaches in sociology which have looked at the social construction of scientific and other knowledges (Nettleton 1992: 133). But is there continuity here? For Foucault, the term 'discourse' referred both to the historically contingent sets of practices (for instance, the practices which constitute clinical medicine) which limit human actions and what may be thought, *and* to the theoretical concept which accounts for the fact that humans actually do act and think in line with these 'regimes of truth' (for instance, that people do – by and large – co-operate with a clinical gaze which turns them into patients). Foucault's archaeological and genealogical accounts address the first of these conceptions of discourse, and it is understandable how these seem attractive to sociologists as explanations of the impact of the social upon how people behave – a central concern of sociology since Durkheim. What seems to follow from this, is a willingness to accept Foucault's theorization of how discourse 'in and of itself' works, as reflected in the sometimes unthinking use of the term in sociology and cognate disciplines. An exploration of this theory of discourse may suggest a more cautious response from sociology.

Foucault sought to develop a basis for understanding what makes knowledge possible, to attempt an 'archaeology' of knowledge, underpinned by 'rules' which operate independently of subjectivity (Foucault 1974: 15–16). As such it has some aspects in common with linguistics, in which a set of grammatical rules authorizes an infinite set of language statements. Thus there is a 'deep' level of rules, and a surface level of discursive statements. Discursive practices are, he says

> characterised by a delimitation of a field of objects, the definition of a legitimate perspective for the agent of knowledge, and the fixing of norms for the elaboration of concepts and theories. (Foucault 1977b: 199)

Three aspects of Foucault's ontology of discourse can be identified. First, while subjects may be capable of interpreting the surface meanings of discursive practices, and thus developing a contingent 'knowledge', the 'deeper' knowledge is not directly accessible, mainly because it is not knowledge at all in the everyday sense of the word. The system of rules which governs the production, operation and regulation of discursive statements (the surface level) mediates *power* or more precisely a 'will to power'. This is not the will of one particular person or group but a generalized will to create the possibilities to be able to 'speak the truth' (Hacking 1986: 34–5). The will to power is productive of new ways of saying plausible things about other human beings and ourselves. Subjectivity (that is, the ability to know oneself) is itself achieved through discourse (as the child of a deeper 'power/knowledge'), clarifying why a prior, privileged or essential subject must be unacceptable within a Foucauldian framework (Nettleton 1992: 131).

Second, Foucault recognizes discursive practices as human activity, 'embodied in technical processes, in institutions, in patterns for general behaviour, in forms for transmission and diffusion, and in pedagogical forms which, at once, impose and maintain them' (Foucault 1977b: 200). However, not all human activity or other events are discursive. Most 'real' historical events or pieces of human behaviour are what Foucault calls 'non-discursive practices', and the relationship between discourse and the non-discursive is not simply a mirroring, in which discourse is the surface manifestation of 'reality' (Brown and Cousins 1986: 36). Rather, discourse is the surface manifestation of the underlying will to power (which Foucault calls 'power/knowledge' in his later work) which cannot be reduced to human intentionality (ibid.: 37–8). Indeed, power/knowledge is that which links discourse to the non-discursive, that creates the connections which makes it possible to speak about some aspect of the world in a particular regime of truth. That which is non-discursive plays no part in such regimes, and whether or not it becomes discursive cannot be determined from essential features of the event itself.

Finally, if power/knowledge is unknowable in a traditional sense, then it follows that no one or no group such as the sovereign, the bourgeoisie or the state can (intentionally) be its author or possess it absolutely (Foucault 1980c: 98). Neither is discourse something which coincides necessarily with single works or groups of works or even specific disciplines. Discourse in this sense has a life of its own independent of human agency (Foucault 1977b: 200–1), and cannot be reduced to particular texts or practices. It is also clear, that given the unknowability of power/knowledge, discerning its 'hidden meaning' could not be the objective of analysis, Foucauldian or otherwise.

This ontology of discourse is quite different from humanist sociological notions of the structuring of agency (Hacking 1986: 35, Smart 1985: 71). To summarize, discourse cannot be reduced to texts or other 'authored' practices, does not directly mirror the 'reality' of historical events (the non-discursive), and is the surface manifestation of a deeper power/knowledge, which is anonymous, disseminated and cannot be known in a traditional sense. Nor is discourse simply a new way of thinking about social structure, which in traditional social theory – however deterministic – can always be 'explained' (as roles, the economic base or whatever): Foucault's conception of discourse is radically divorced, both from 'reality' and from traditional notions of human subjectivity. It follows that strategies appropriate to a humanistic framework, for instance recourse to authorial intention, historical events or contexts, cannot be adopted when utilizing this model.

The unfamiliarity of such a notion of an ahistorical, non-authored discourse governed by a free-floating, anonymous, disseminated power/

knowledge requires most cautious methodological rigour when applied to sociological analysis. Two opposing attractors await the unwary, and examples of both are discernible in the work of Foucauldian sociologists.

The first of these is a tendency for essentialism concerning power/knowledge, such that power is seen as unitary and unifying, working through disciplinary discourses to achieve its ends. This can be seen most clearly in neo-Marxist or structuralist analyses, in which power is 'functional', closely associated with the interests of some group or institution (Wickham 1986: 153, 170–4). The second tendency leads in the opposite direction, to a position in which power/knowledge is acknowledged as unknowable and thus either vacuous (Rorty 1992: 330) or simply to be quietly forgotten about altogether, in favour of a focus on the surface phenomenon of discursive practice.

Foucault was aware of how easy it would be to essentialize power (Freundlieb 1994: 158–62), but argued this would be to undermine his perspective on it as strategic, rather than something to be possessed, such that

> its effects of domination are attributed not to 'appropriation', but to dispositions, manoeuvres, tactics, techniques, functionings; that one should decipher in it a network of relations constantly in tension, in activity ... that one should take as its model a perpetual battle rather than a contract regulating a transaction or the conquest of a territory. (Foucault 1979: 26)

At the level of the rules governing discourse, power/knowledge was a principle of 'dispersion' rather than a unity (Freundlieb 1994: 162), and was located between rather than within institutions (Foucault 1979: 26). Despite this pronouncement, Wickham (1986: 152–7) does discern occasions in which power/knowledge come over as unitary and prior in Foucault's own writing, and it is unsurprising that from time to time a notion of power as something which is wilful and can 'use' discourse emerges in Foucauldian studies. So, for example, Armstrong writes that

> Panoptic power had fabricated bodies by making them the objects of an observing eye. The new regime exercised surveillance over the whole population and, because it observed the mind of everyone, was in a better position to make the individual a point of articulation for power: both an effect of power and a point from which power was exercised. (Armstrong 1983: 70)

Similarly, Sawicki reflects on Foucauldian notions of power, asking

> If patriarchal power operated primarily through violence, objectifica-
> tion and repression, why would women subject themselves to it
> willingly? On the other hand, if it also operates by inciting desire,
> attaching individuals to specific identities, and addressing real needs,
> then it is easier to understand how it has been so effective at getting a
> grip on us. (Sawicki 1991: 85)

At the extreme, power/knowledge becomes synonymous with 'the state'
or 'society' or some particular grouping, reflecting a functionalism which
can sometimes be discerned in *Discipline and Punish* (Donnelly 1986: 29,
Hoy 1986: 7–8). For example, Maseide describes a 'control model' to
describe how 'adequate' clinical practice is achieved by doctors.

> Power is thought of as always necessary to the clinical encounter, and
> in that respect often benign. It enables the doctor to act as situationally
> and institutionally competent. Such competence is often demanded by
> patients and it is legally and professionally prescribed. ... Power is made
> effective through forms of control and methods of domination. ... As
> such, they are essential resources for the doctor's ability to do his or her
> clinical work adequately. ... The impact of power is effective to the
> extent that doctor and patient share a system of knowledge and
> assumptions that facilitates relatively conflict-free interaction and effec-
> tive patient compliance. (Maseide 1991: 552–3)

Here the relations of power are brought into such close allegiance with the
grouping in whose interest power works (that is, the medical profession)
that we are back with sovereign (essential) power (Wickham 1986: 171–2).

If this first tendency brings back human agency through the back door,
by essentializing power/knowledge as unitary, sovereign and thus potentially the possession of a person or persons, the second reintroduces
humanism elsewhere: through the authorial voice of the texts which
contribute to discourse. Foucault became less concerned with the *archaeology* of the 'rules' of discursive formation, as with the *genealogy* of
power/knowledge: the changing relationship of discourse to the non-
discursive over time (Smart 1985: 42), in other words to the objects of
history – in particular, bodies, selves and subjectivity in general.

Foucault's genealogies draw more heavily on the surface manifestations
of discursive practices, the human productions of texts or non-textual
practices. There is thus the potential for any text or practice to be labelled

'discursive', eliding the distinction between written texts and 'discourse', between which Foucault quite clearly differentiates (Foucault 1977a: 123, 138; 1977b: 200). Genealogy supplies apparently convincing analyses of historical changes in discursive practices, filled with examples drawn from the surface manifestations. The existence of a discourse is discerned inductively, and with enough ingenuity any text can be linked to a 'discourse'. To give two examples: firstly, Paden's exploration of Puritan writings since the fifth century discerns the development of a reflexive identity, such that he concludes:

> Puritan writing, in spite of its God-centred theology, not only presupposed the importance of the self, the 'seeing I', but also pre-figured the modern division of the self into opposing parts. ... Puritan suspicion of self represented a practice with implications which go well beyond the mythological agenda that invented it. By the logic of reflexive self-examination, every religious assertion ... could become subject of its own possible self-deception. (Paden 1988: 78)

Similarly, having documented various Victorian texts which reported studies of the association of sugar with dental decay, Nettleton suggests that

> Each of these studies with their various and often conflicting conclusions was an attempt to find the 'truth' about the relationship between sugar and caries. But there was a more fundamental truth which each of these studies has already presumed, namely the existence of mouths, teeth, sugar and disease. ... In effect, arguments for and against (sugar's) value were all part of the same discourse. (Nettleton 1992: 81)

Such studies are based in the Foucauldian premise that the rules of discursive formation provide the 'conditions of existence' of particular statements, which make it possible to say certain things and not others: the 'discourse' is inductively derived from the texts under study. But what precisely is happening here? In Foucault's position, discourse is anonymous, dependent neither on human intent nor historical context, and cannot be reduced to the texts of specific 'authors' (Foucault 1977a: 121), yet genealogy concerns itself principally with texts, from which we 'uncover' the discourse. Freundlieb suggests (1994: 176) that behind such analysis is a 'hidden model of historical sociology' which links discursive practices to historical events (non-discursive practices) in precisely the way which Foucault rejected. Capitalism, industrial development, the physicality of the body, particular historical events or whatever form an unacknowledged backcloth which structures the analytical work of discerning the 'rules' of discursive formation. Reflecting on Foucault's own strategy for linking the non-discursive to the discursive, Freundlieb rather cynically comments that

> all the examples Foucault provides of changes in discursive formations simply name singular historical events. In other word, each so-called rule he postulates only applies once, thus emptying the notion of a rule of all content. (ibid.: 171)

Transposed to sociology, it has been argued that Foucault's approach can 'rehabilitate' structuralist and functionalist kinds of analysis which de-emphasize agency, by rejecting the concept of 'sovereign' power and thus overcoming the determinism of such analyses (Silverman 1985). In this section I have suggested that while Foucault's theorizing of discourse enabled him to construct quasi-historical accounts of regimes of truth, it does not work so well within a sociological application. On one hand, his version of discourse can result in a highly deterministic and essentialist reading of power (Lupton 1997: 102), while on the other, genealogies may turn out to depend far more upon authorial intent than is admitted. These tendencies towards determinism and humanism will be revisited in the next two sections.

The Foucauldian Ontology of Body

In his effort to avoid the 'liberal conception of individuals as uncon-strained, creative essences' (Wickham 1986: 15), Foucault chose in works such as *Birth of the Clinic* and *Discipline and Punish* to deprivilege ration-ality and focus on the body as the site and target of power. This was indeed an effective rhetorical device for destabilizing some of the assump-tions of philosophical discourse, opening up new ways of thinking 'subject', 'power' and 'knowledge'. Furthermore, it was central to the generation of genealogies of institutional power. Genealogy, Foucault suggested, is a strategy which seeks to account for the constitution of knowledge from within the flow of history, rather than by reference to some supposedly objective standpoint such as 'madness' or 'criminality' (Foucault 1986: 59).

The genealogical approach, primarily a strategy to critique issues in philosophy and history, has gained the attention of sociologists concerned with issues of embodiment, notably in the sociologies of health, gender and sexuality. However, the emergence of a 'sociology of the body' (Turner

1992, Nettleton 1995) raises problems for this ontology. Firstly, by making the 'body' the new privileged object of a sociology, a new essentialism beckons, in which the body becomes the pre-existing focus of power's action, in place of a 'self', an 'individual' or an 'agent'. There is the potential for this Foucauldian body to become a romantic subject-substitute, continually buffeted by discourse, never able to self-actualize, doomed always to be the plaything of power/knowledge (Hacking 1986: 28). On the other hand, one has to question whether the ontological (or non-ontological) status attributed to the body by Foucault is really adequate for a 'sociology of the body'; one is led to ask: *which* body?

1. The body is the physical body. For the strict Foucauldian, such a position is not acceptable. While from the early pages of *Discipline and Punish* (Foucault 1979), it might be concluded that the physical body is the focus of disciplinary power, throughout that work, and in his *Birth of the Clinic*, Foucault argues that power does not act directly on some biological entity (1976: x). Indeed, the concept of the biological body, the 'organism' or 'body-with-organs' (Deleuze and Guattari 1988: 158) is itself discursively constructed – by theology, by philosophy, by biomedicine and other discourses.

2. It is some kind of 'natural body' underpinning the 'organism'. Those who shy away from 'radical constructionism' (Nettleton 1995: 29), and acknowledge a natural body which is overlaid with cultural values, adopt an essentialist position, albeit one in which the essence's existence is determined phenomenologically, through 'experience', faith or 'common sense' (see, for example, Collins 1994). This position has been adopted in some post-structuralist feminisms, which while taking on board the perspective of the body as discursively constructed, wish at the same time to recognize the specific experience of sexual difference (McNay 1992: 36).

3. There is some kind of 'natural' body, but it is beyond discourse and thus unknowable. This avoids the tag of essentialism, but leaves us with a meaningless and pointless construct. As such, the 'sociology of the body' becomes the 'sociology of ?'.

4. It is always already some kind of socially constructed body and it is 'impossible to know the materiality of the body outside its cultural significations' (McNay 1992: 30). While there are certain actions and gestures in physical space, certain states of mind within the brain,

anything which can be called a unified 'body' is the creation of power/knowledge. This Foucauldian body – a 'Body-without-Organs' (Deleuze and Guattari 1984, 1988) is a social body throughout.

While there may be a willingness on the part of some sociologists of the body to indulge in 'epistemological pragmatism' (Turner 1992: 61), choosing from the alternatives above as the task in hand requires, for the Foucauldian protagonist of the 'sociology of the body', the phrase must surely be ironic, referring to the disappearance (or appearance?) of 'the body' as it is discursively written. Foucault himself seemed entirely unconcerned about whatever kind of material entity the body might be, and the way he wrote of the body implied that he often did not have in mind a conventional notion of the body at all. For example, using the Deleuzian term 'phantasms' to describe the writing of the body by discourse, he wrote that

> Phantasms must be allowed to function at the limit of bodies; against bodies, because they stick to bodies and protrude from them, but also because they touch them, cut them, break them into sections, regionalise them, and multiply their surfaces, and equally outside of bodies, because they function between bodies. (1977c: 169–70)

For Foucault, the important thing was not the body itself, but that it was both realized in the play of power and also the site of possible transgressions or refusals of power (Game 1991: 45). Civilization as the project of history relentlessly writes this body, seeking its total destruction by its transfiguration into a cultural object (Butler 1990: 129–30). This formulation reveals another aspect of the determinism of Foucault's ontology. Foucault's version of the body, despite his obvious political and personal inclinations to be on the side of those who are resistant (Haber 1994), turns out to be 'totally imprinted by discourse' (Butler 1990), and 'passive and largely deprived of causal powers' (Lash 1991: 261–70). Foucault's analysis worked well in circumstances where discursive regimes of truth were successful in constructing relatively unresisting subjectivities, for example, the sick and the mentally ill. But such a model cannot analyse the conditions under which resistance to power becomes possible, why some people resist and others do not, and how resistance may be successful – all issues of great interest to sociologists from Marx through Goffman to Bauman. Furthermore, although the model may be a useful tool for analysis, it cannot be a catalyst for resistance (Haber 1994: 111): while resistance is always an aspect of power (Foucault 1980a: 142), to codify resistance is to destroy it.

The passiveness of such a non-embodied body comes across in some sociological writing. Lupton (1997) chides Armstrong for his determinism, and we can find many examples of similar reification. Thus, Harding's discussion of hormone replacement therapy (HRT) and the construction of the female body concludes that

> HRT can be viewed as a technology of power directed at bodies which establishes, at the level of the body, unequal distributions of power and thereby contributes to the manufacture of sexed subjects and the definition of conditions of being a sex. Sex can be seen as an effect of the investments in the body made possible by discourses, in this case on HRT, producing its natural and normal precondition and subsequent secondary characterisations. (1997: 147)

By denying any essential self, such analyses leave the non-discursive physical body entirely divorced from the discursive body written by power/knowledge. Such a position has seemed unsatisfactory to many sociologists; to post-structuralist feminists – whose agenda is both analytical and political – in particular. Sawicki sees the subjectification of women by discourses on reproduction as creating possibilities for resistance to patriarchy, for example, through demands for infertility treatment by lesbians and single women (Sawicki 1991: 84). Butler warns that Foucault seems to be adhering to a long and suspect tradition in which the body is the passive recipient of culture, proposing instead a body whose performative gender identity can resist and subvert (Butler 1990: 129, 141). Annandale and Clark more bluntly argue that

> the body, as a hinge term constituted through social relations, is both culture and nature ... In both creating and being transformed by culture, the body as culture and nature is by the same token both sex and gender. (1996)

The inadequacy of this Foucauldian ontology of the body for some sociological tasks – to be an interface between different domains – biological and social, collective and individual, constrained and free (Bertholet 1991: 398), has led some sociologists to turn to other works by Foucault for a more congenial model.

The Foucauldian Ontology of Self

Once engaged on his project concerning human sexuality, Foucault's work underwent a refocusing away from the body, toward 'the self'. This move,

Foucault suggested, represented a 'shift' of emphasis (Foucault 1985: 6) to establish an analysis complementary to his earlier studies of knowledge and power, although to some it appeared as

> a tacit admission by Foucault that his previous work, which so systematically attacked and undermined the notion of the subject, had been along the wrong lines and had run itself into a theoretical dead end. (McNay 1992: 48)

Can this 'return of the subject' successfully address the sociological need for a more subtle ontology which can theorize resistance? The ontological problem concerning resistance was one which Foucault was to acknowledge (often with great poignancy) in many later interviews (for example Martin 1988), and as he laboured to construct an ethics of the self, he wrote of individuals not as docile bodies but as reflexive, living, speaking beings (Foucault 1985: 7). The reflexive self theorized in the volumes of the *History of Sexuality* contributes a more active notion of subjectivity, in place of the passive bodies of the earlier carceral model (McNay 1992: 49–50). A living, speaking, reflexive subjectivity implies the capacity to resist, and Foucault (1977c: 165) appeared to endorse Deleuze's theorizing of a mechanism by which such an active subject may actively interpret and rewrite discourse and hence its own subjectivity (Lash 1991: 264–6).

In this writing, 'individual', and 'self' supplement the more usual 'subject' and 'body'; in his writing on the *History of Sexuality* (Foucault 1984, 1985, 1986, 1988b) the move from concern with external technologies of power to technologies of the self is clear. Now Foucault's project is with how we become 'desiring subjects', in other words, how we articulate our bodies and desires within a subjectivity capable of reflection. 'Practices of the self' mark the engagement between discourses of the social and the individual, such that power is integral to the autonomous ordering of individuals' own lives (McNay 1992: 67). Personal identities emerge not as prior and privileged ontologically, but 'in a battlefield', in which difference and opposition are the means by which identity and the boundaries of others become discernible (Pizzorno 1992: 207). This formulation overcomes the criticism of Foucault's ontology which leaves individuals as passive and totally inscribed by discourse, for now it can be seen that reflexivity plays a crucial part in the process of subjectivity. Yet the ontological implications of Foucault's later position need further scrutiny, and three issues have been raised by critics, which are highly relevant for the application of the position in the social analysis of health and health care.

First, Foucault's ontology of the body has subtly changed. In *Power/Knowledge* (Foucault 1980a–d), he speaks of something which escapes power, which is an 'inverse energy', a 'discharge', 'energies and irreducibilities'. As in Deleuze and Guattari (1984), resistance is predicated upon this notion of something beyond and irreducible to discourse: a position in apparent contradiction to all that has gone before concerning the relationship between discourse and the non-discursive (Hoy 1986: 8, Pizzorno 1992: 207, Wickham 1986). Such positions would imply, in terms of the earlier evaluation of how the body is to be understood, a move from category four (a totally cultural body) to category two, in which the body is 'natural' in some way, but overlaid with cultural values.

We can see this reflected in some of the sociological writings that have taken this position. The Krokers' analysis of sexuality in the postmodern era speaks of '... bodies living on their own borrowed power; violent and alternating, scenes of surplus energy and perfect inertness ...' (Kroker and Kroker 1988: 22), and Sawicki suggests that technologies mobilize bodies, not by violence but, *inter alia* by '... inciting and channelling desires, generating and focusing individual and group energies' (Sawicki 1991: 83).

Second, by emphasizing the autonomy of the individual, within a governmentality which leads to a relativist 'art of existence' (that is, a reflexive and contextualized sense of what it means to be a self), Foucault's 'techniques of the self' are reduced to 'self stylizations'. These fail to differentiate between practices that are merely 'suggested' to the individual, and practices that are more or less 'imposed' in so far as they are heavily laden with cultural sanctions and taboos (McNay 1992: 74). Governmentality seems to offer such a degree of autonomy to the individual that it effectively shifts the balance from Foucault's earlier determinism concerning the 'rules' which determine which practices become discursive, to a relatively autonomous subjectivity. In a sociological context, the position might end up looking much like a phenomenological account. Thus Weedon argues that

> (a)lthough the subject in post-structuralism is socially constructed in discursive practices, she none the less exists as a thinking, feeling subject and social agent, capable of resistance and innovations produced out of the clash between different contradictory subject positions and practices. She is also a subject able to reflect upon the discursive relations which constitute her and the society in which she lives, and able to choose from the options available. (1987: 125)

Similarly, in Eckermann's analysis of self-starvation, those who starve themselves may move from self-effacement to self-embracing, to 'recreate a sense of self' through their new body shape (Eckermann 1997: 166–7).

Third, it was noted earlier that genealogy focuses for its raw material on texts, as in Foucault's final writings on sexuality. Poster argues that, whereas in such works as *Discipline and Punish* Foucault could interpret Bentham's texts on the Panopticon in ways which turned the author's intentions on their heads (1986: 217), *The Care of the Self* is closer to a traditional history of ideas, relying heavily upon the intentional level of meaning and explicit phrases of 'key' textual accounts (for example, the writings of Plato or Marcus Aurelius). We saw how sociologists such as Paden and Nettleton have adopted a genealogical approach, and they, alongside Foucault himself, are open to traditional criticisms concerning the justification of precisely which texts are 'key'. Both Poster (ibid.: 218) and McNay (1992: 77–9) have offered alternative explanations to Foucault's efforts to interpret historical notions of sexuality, such as ancient Greek attitudes to sexual overindulgence. 'Discourse' has become a moveable feast.

Taken together, these shifts of emphasis undermine most aspects of the earlier positions concerning discourse and its relation to the non-discursive. The non-discursive 'residue' enables resistance to power/knowledge, no doubt providing a resource to the reflexive self as it is inscribed by discourse, while such subjects contribute to the generation of discourse through their texts. From what might be seen as an overemphasis on determinism, we now find an overemphasis on agency. Rorty has suggested that Foucault's dilemma rested on his twin aspirations – to be both a moral citizen concerned with the possibilities for resistance to power, and his refusal to be complicit with power by taking on its own vocabulary of essentialized subjects (Rorty 1992: 330–1). While his work on power and truth met the latter objective at the expense of the former, the reintroduction of a self privileges the former but makes his previous ontology untenable. Unfortunately both positions are naive when applied in sociology, and the much-vaunted *rapprochement* of agency and structure is illusory.

Beyond Foucault

I have tried in these sections to unpack elements of Foucault's theorizing of discourse, power and subjectivity, and to show how these are frequently strained in Foucauldian sociology, both because of the multiple threads running through Foucault's own work, and because of the different concerns of history, philosophy and sociology. The question which has to be asked in this concluding section is whether sociology should 'forget Foucault', to use Baudrillard's phrase. Foucault's frame of reference rewrites human subjects in ways which challenge humanist understandings of self and others, and some sociologists may choose to live with the ambiguities and contradictions outlined here for the sake of the novelty of accounts generated by the approach. Others might argue that ambiguity and contradiction are a feature of any enterprise which seeks to persuade (Derrida 1978), and that as such, are particularly suited to a postmodern sociology. I can see some justification in both these positions, and I will spend a little time looking at each before coming to my own position concerning Foucault's contribution to sociology.

First, it is certainly the case that Foucault's work is both appealing to the sociological imagination, combining as it apparently does the attractions of both structuralist approaches and social constructionism, *and* offering the promise of novel accounts. Within the sociology of health and illness, Foucault's *Birth of the Clinic* spawned a generation of archaeology/ genealogy, with writers such as Armstrong working their way through the pantheon of medical specialties. Like the earlier *Madness and Civilisation,* Foucault's study of clinical medicine was highly criticized as inaccurate and fanciful within historical circles (Armstrong 1997: 20), but that is less of a problem for sociologists. Foucault has given sociology a way of writing history which links the innovation of technologies or ideas with the cultural context in which they arise (ibid.), a position held in common with the 'strong programme' sociologists of scientific knowledge (Bloor 1976). This elision of quite different theoretical frameworks (Fox 1993a: 151) may have led to the tendency to use the term 'discourse' as a shorthand for any kind of proposition, and – as was noted in the discussion of 'sociological genealogies' – the inclination to treat all texts as 'discursive' regardless of their status or relationship with other texts. Such studies have little or nothing in common with Foucault's own methods of analysis.

Foucault's work also appeals to the political imagination within sociology, offering a model of power less monolithic than those of either Marx or Weber. Indeed the panopticon, whose gaze is the key central to both *Birth of the Clinic* and *Discipline and Punish,* subtly rereads the Weberian analysis of the rationalizations of capitalism which set the scene for the era of modernity (Fox 1991). What for Weber was an iron cage of regulation and law, for Foucault becomes an open prison committed to abolishing the last dark corner in which the soul might hide, and yet in which resistance is ubiquitous, a function of power as much as the gaze itself. Particularly within feminist sociology, this position has been highly productive, although as has been shown in this chapter, on occasions this scholarship cuts across fundamentals of Foucault's positions concerning subjectivity and 'empowerment' in its challenge to patriarchy. In hands less skilled than Foucault's own, efforts to use the Foucauldian notion of the self come to look much like phenomenological sociology.

The second justification for the use of Foucauldian or quasi-Foucauldian approaches might consist in an argument for a postmodern, fragmentary social theory, accepting of paradox and contradiction, and committed to opening up new readings rather than seeking truth in a definitive account (Owen 1997). From such a perspective, the kinds of problems with using Foucault in sociology which this chapter has illus-trated are not problems at all, but features of the end of a modernist meta-narrative for sociology. The structure/agency dichotomy is not resolved by Foucault, rather it is seen as incapable of resolution: and ceases to be a problem. Foucauldian genealogies can proliferate, and even those which are contradictory in their analyses can coexist: Foucault's role now becomes that of an unsettler, reminding us that social science is itself part of the history of ideas. Yet Foucault is actually a bad candidate for this kind of sociology, given the extent to which his work itself constitutes a kind of meta-narrative (Nettleton 1995), typified – according to Mouzelis (1995) – by vagueness, grandiosity and overgeneralization.

While I have sympathy with a political project to destabilize sociology's modernist project (as perhaps would Foucault, given his analysis of the human sciences in *The Order of Things*), my own appraisal of the Foucauldian corpus is different. Indeed, Foucault has contributed to the post-structuralist movements of the late second millennium which have radicalized the agendas of philosophy, literary theory and emancipatory politics. However, I believe the translation of Foucault into sociology is largely vapid, except to the extent that philosophy, literary theory and emancipatory politics impinge on the discipline. In this chapter I have sought to show its limitations: firstly, that the kinds of questions the disci-pline asks are much wider than those within Foucault's project; secondly, that the 'tools' he created won't work beyond these limits; and thirdly, that when adapted by Foucauldians so they do appear to work, the methods are indistinguishable from more traditional approaches.

For these reasons, I have been forced to abandon any efforts to use Foucault's theory in my efforts to theorize resistance, and to explore how it might be possible to move *beyond* health. Already in this book, I have used the work of Derrida, Lyotard, Cixous and others to develop my position. All these writers have explored the issue of power, and all have identified ways of resisting that power. For example, Derrida's theory of *différance* suggests that undecidability limits the impact of any regime of power. For Cixous, *écriture feminine* is a means of rethinking the world which – for her – suggests how masculine power may be resisted. Together, these and other post-structuralist writers have developed a body of theory which can inform the modelling of a non-essentialist, resisting subject engaged within a 'politics of difference' (Haber 1994). In the next chapter, I shall develop the perspective which I have found the most helpful in thinking about how we might move *beyond* health: the nomadology of Deleuze and Guattari.

5
Deleuze, Guattari and the Politics of Embodiment

When Deleuze and Guattari (1984, 1988) wrote of a 'Body-without-Organs' (henceforth, BwO), they supplied cultural and social theory with a powerful concept for understanding the cultural inscription of human beings' bodies, minds and souls. As I shall show, the BwO is quite unlike the 'organism' or 'body-with-organs' which religion, law and biomedicine have hegemonized in our common-sense understanding of embodiment. The BwO is a philosophical surface upon which the social plays, establishing a reflexivity in its subject-matter While the BwO is the site of domination, it is also the site of resistance and refusal. As such it is a locus of a micropolitics, and what Deleuze and Guattari call a 'nomadology' (Deleuze and Guattari 1988).

In this chapter I shall trace this micropolitical BwO through readings of Deleuze and Guattari's work, as might be seen through the lenses of Derrida on knowledge and the margin, Haraway on the cyborg, Kristeva and Cixous on intertextuality and the rewriting of the self. This fragmenting and disembodying supplies the key to the argument of this book, about what it means to move *beyond* health.

The French philosopher Gilles Deleuze established an intellectual partnership with the psychoanalyst Felix Guattari shortly after the May 1968 revolt by students and workers in Paris. Timing is relevant, because May '68 was an event which – in retrospect, at least – was emblematic for the trends in Francophone philosophy critical of both capitalism and state socialism, as reflected in the works of Derrida, Foucault, Lyotard and others discussed in this book. Deleuze and Guattari's collaboration continued until the 1990s and was ended by the death of Guattari, to be followed shortly afterwards by Deleuze's own demise. The corpus of their shared authorship includes the major works *Anti-Oedipus* (1984), *A Thousand Plateaus* (1988) and *What is Philosophy?* (1994).

In common with a range of other post-structuralist French writers, the works of Deleuze and Guattari have been slow to impact within Anglo sociology, their influence to date being strongest within cultural studies and political sociology (Braidotti 1993, Patton 1995). So in the coming pages I shall introduce the principal concepts in Deleuze and Guattari's writing, and suggest how these might be applied to elucidate the themes and problems with which I am concerned.

Before that, it is worth situating Deleuze and Guattari within an intellectual framework. Born in 1925 and a student of philosophy in 1940s Paris, Deleuze's influences – like those of others such as Foucault and Derrida who were to rise to prominence in French philosophy in the 1970s and '80s – included Nietzsche, Bergson and Heidegger, and resulted in such works as *Difference and Repetition* (1968) and *The Logic of Sense* (1969). While this anti-rationalist tradition coincided with French structuralism's emphasis on the centrality of language in constructing both the world and the self, he was critical of structuralist ontology as impersonal and overdeterministic (Bogue 1989: 2–3). An associate of Foucault's, he wrote an interesting study of that writer's work (Deleuze 1988) which is both a discussion of Foucault and of Deleuze's own take on the issues with which Foucault concerned himself.

Guattari was born in 1930 and following studies in pharmacy and philosophy became involved in oppositional politics, both as a member of the French Communist Party and in challenges to tradition models of mental illness and its treatment. During the 1960s he underwent psychoanalysis with Lacan and subsequently became a Lacanian analyst. However, it was his rejection of Lacan's blend of Freud and Saussurian structuralism, in favour of an effort to synthesize Freud and Marx, which provided the basis for his association with Deleuze (Bogue 1989: 5–6). For both Deleuze and Guattari, the collaboration over their first joint work, *Anti-Oedipus* (published in France in 1972, and sub-titled *Capitalism and Schizophrenia*) may be seen as synergistic from earlier (though different) commitments and intellectual influences, and as an innovative direction which was to be developed over the following decade.

In the next sections, I will examine three of Deleuze and Guattari's concepts which are of particular relevance to the resisting subject: the Body-without-Organs, territorialization and nomadology). However, there is not space here for more than a summary of Deleuze and Guattari's project in *Anti-Oedipus* and readers are referred to the work itself and to exegeses such as Bogue (1989), Massumi (1992) or Fox (1993a) for fuller accounts. *Anti-Oedipus*, and to an extent its companion work *A Thousand Plateaus*, are challenges to the Lacanian view of desire, the key concept in psychoanalysis to explain human motivation and psychodynamics. Freud and Freudians such as Lacan considered desire as subverted by the Oedipus conflict into attachments which led to neurosis. The task of psycho-analysis was to expose the displacements or condensations by which these undesirable attachments had become established and to refocus desire upon more appropriate targets.

In *Anti-Oedipus*, Deleuze and Guattari criticize Lacan's 'linguistic Freudianism' for its elaboration of a conception of desire as always to be understood as a lack or absence of an object (food, the mother, the lover, the phallus etc.), and as part of the realm of the psyche which Freud called the *symbolic*, and thus distanced from the 'real' world which impinges on the human subject. Because this desire is symbolic, it is bound to fail, because it cannot possess its (real) object. As Butler (1990) comments, this leads to what Nietzsche called a 'slave mentality', and Deleuze and Guattari argue that what sustains this slavishness are the social relations of capitalism and the family form. Their critique of psychoanalysis is thus part of an antagonism to 'state philosophy' (Massumi 1992: 4–5) – the co-option or mutual constitution of nation-state and philosophy from ancient Greece to the modern period (Deleuze and Guattari 1994: 103ff). The possibility of an alternative to this philosophy of identity and control is a thread running through both Deleuze's early work and his collabora-tion with Guattari, and made most explicit in *What is Philosophy?* (Deleuze and Guattari 1994).

Deleuze and Guattari do not deny the existence of this Lacanian/ Freudian symbolic desire-as-lack, but propose in addition a conception of positive desire which is both real and productive, a creative affirmation of potential (Massumi 1992: 174) akin to Nietzsche's will-to-power of the organism (Bogue 1989: 23–4). By the exertion of this will-to-power, it is possible for the human subject to be active rather than reactive, to meet its (real) needs and free itself from the chains of oppression under capi-talism. They attack psychoanalysis for denying the possibility of such engagement with the world, for making a virtue of refocusing an individ-ual's desire on the *symbolic* Oedipal *Mother–Father–Ego* triad. This, in Deleuze and Guattari's view, is a pathological symptom of the capitalist commodification of the world and its contents as objects to be possessed.

The importance of Deleuze and Guattari's emphasis on human beings' will to power or affirmation of potential is developed in their follow-up work *A Thousand Plateaus* (also sub-titled *Capitalism and Schizophrenia*), which focuses less on the ills of psychoanalysis and more on the process of resisting oppression (Massumi 1992: 82). In the latter work, what is implied by these concepts is that human beings are active and motivated rather than passive, and incorporative of their engagement with the world through an on-going work of sense-making. It is this aspect of Deleuze and Guattari's model which is of greatest relevance for this book: that the construction of subjectivity is in the *dialogical* play of social processes and the affirmative and active creation of meaning (the will-to-power) as the human being engages with the world.

Readers may at this point recognize the crucial difference from the Foucauldian perspective which I was at pains to explore in the last chapter. Foucault's ontology denies the activity of the subject; for him subjectivity is simply the play of power/knowledge on a passive substrate. It is to describe the *constructive* act of selfhood that Deleuze and Guattari introduce the notions of the Body-without-Organs, of the territorialization of this entity by the social, and of nomadology as the strategic resistance of territorialization. The rest of this chapter is devoted to exploring these ideas, and how they inform a politics of disembodiment.

The Body-without-Organs

> The full body without organs is the unproductive, the sterile, the unengendered, the unconsumable. (Deleuze and Guattari 1984: 8)

Anti-Oedipus, with its polemical style, is not necessarily the best place to start to explore the relevance and utility of the notion of the BwO. This term can be traced back to Deleuze's earlier book *The Logic of Sense* (1969, 1990), in which he coined the terminology in homage to Artaud's description of being without shape or form during catatonic schizophrenia. Deleuze and Guattari (1984: 9) quote Artaud thus 'The body is the body/it is all by itself/and has no need of organs/the body is never an organism/organisms are the enemy of the body'. This phenomenology was part of Deleuze's intellectual commitment to explicate the relationship between reality and meaning without recourse to an essential subjectivity, and the collaborative work of Deleuze and Guattari which applies the concept of the BwO can be seen as an extension of this project. In *Anti-Oedipus* (which – as was noted earlier – was written as a diatribe against Lacanian psychoanalysis), the term becomes the pivotal relation between the subjective sense-of-self and the social environment. The BwO is decidedly not the physical body:

> The body without organs is not the proof of an original nothingness, nor is it what remains of a lost totality. Above all, it is not a projection; it has nothing whatsoever to do with the body itself or with an image

of the body. It is the body without an image. (Deleuze and Guattari
1984: 8)

Rather it is the metaphorical or metaphysical 'surface' which links (and
allows the interpenetration of) psychic experience with the forces of
society. By means of this concept they establish a connection between the
realms of the psychological and the social, between Freud and Marx. The
BwO is the surface, that is the psychical locus, upon which are inscribed
and recorded all the forces of capitalist production, such that '... the schizo
practises political economy, and all sexuality is a matter of economy'
(Deleuze and Guattari 1984: 12). In *The Logic of Sense*, Deleuze sought to
analyse how the collision of the forces of the social (conceived by Deleuze
as the forces of capitalist production) with the organism's will-to-power (or
positive desire) creates sense-of-self, and furthermore, of how it is possible
to resist such social forces. It is from this wider reading that we can see the
relevance of the notion of the BwO to issues of embodiment, health and
illness.

The Body-without-Organs is important for my analysis because it is
developed within an anti-essentialist framework – there is no prior 'essence'
of self. Yet while acknowledging the construction of self (and thereby, the
body) as a continuing project of the social, it is understood as a dynamic
rather than a passive process of 'inscription'. Thus we can recognize the
impact of the social world on how we understand our selves and our bodies,
for example, in the kinds of analyses developed by Foucault and his
followers, critically examined in chapter 4. Power, mediated through
systems of thought and knowledge, instigates a reflexive sense-of-self in its
subjects. At different periods in history, people come to understand their
humanity or selfhood in ways appropriate to the systems of thought of the
day. Just as the body is disciplined (by education, law, medicine etc.), so
subjectivity is disciplined by systems of knowledge – from ancient philosophy and religion to the modern social sciences.

Yet this construction of bodies and selves is not a simple matter of
inscribing a blank sheet. For Deleuze and Guattari, there is a constant
tension between the forces of the social and the BwO's will-to-power. They
describe the construction process as a *territorialization* and thus the BwO
may be thought of as a *territory* constantly contested and fought over. In a
moment I will look at this in more detail, but first, I shall provide an
example of this anti-essentialist way of thinking about embodiment.

Humanistic sociology, with its roots in symbolic interactionism and
phenomenology, is predicated upon an essentialist conception of the
human subject as prior: the entity which experiences, makes sense of, and

thereby has a hand in constructing the social world around it. While some studies in the essentialist tradition have addressed pain, as a topic it has not featured greatly in sociological writing on health and illness, perhaps because it is a 'private sensation' (Baszanger 1992: 181), and has thus appeared 'non-social' in character. From an essentialist perspective, pain – seen as a physiological precursor – is ascribed its meaning by its sufferers, and interest focuses upon the existential circumstances of embodiment which derive from such experience. Thus, for example, Radley (1989) investigates 'adjustment style' among sufferers from chronic pain, while Charmaz suggests that

> (p)hysical pain, psychological distress, and the deleterious effects of medical procedures all cause the chronically ill to suffer as they experience their illness. However, a narrow medicalised view of suffering ignores or minimises the broader significance of suffering: the *loss of self* felt by many people with chronic illnesses. Chronically ill people frequently experience a crumbling away of their former self-images without simultaneous development of equally valued new ones. (Charmaz 1983: 168, emphasis in original)

Deleuze and Guattari's theoretical framework offers an alternative to this essentialist reading, in which there is not a prior, 'interior' self to experience bodily pain. Essentialism, Butler (1990) argues, achieves privilege for the self through this use of metaphors of depth and surface. For Deleuze and Guattari, such oppositions are swept away: the anatomical body is not the carapace of the self, rather, the self which experiences an interiority does so because of a way of thinking (a *territorialization*) which creates a sense of being 'inside' the body. Part of this territorialization is into what Deleuze and Guattari (1988: 158) call the 'organism' or the *'body-with-organs'*, which ascribes meaning to bodily sensation according to systems of thought which in the modern world are dominated by biomedicine.

Pain as sensation has no implicit meaning. But a territorialization of the BwO as organism (creature of biomedical and more recently human sciences discourses) provides the possibility for pain to signify. Once it signifies in relation to the organism, it contributes to the subjectivity which has been territorialized on the BwO. In this reading, it is not the self which experiences pain or attributes meaning to it, the self *is* the pain, the self is an effect of the meaning (Fox 1993a: 145).

A number of studies of pained people suggest the impact upon subjectivity. In de Swaan's (1990) study of a cancer ward, the meanings attached to pain and its significance as marker of finitude and dissolution territorialize not only patients but also relatives and staff. The emotions associated with pain (fear, anger, scorn, panic among others) create a subjectivity which seems to dominate everything else. Subjectivities of a deeply discredited kind (the 'felt stigma' of Scambler and Hopkins 1986), become attached to patients as they are constituted as demented or incapable of following codes of decorum (de Swaan 1990: 53–4). In Perakyla's study of terminal care of patients, hospice models of care constitute an 'experiencing subject' whose suffering can be organized within the systems of care available in the setting. Within a 'psychological frame', motives are imputed to patients which explain their anger or resistance to treatment regimes. By adducing psychological suffering, it supplies an acceptable subjectivity to a patient whose non-compliance might otherwise be stigmatized as deviant (1989: 122–3).

In contrast with such essentialist conceptions of the self, which bemoan the 'biographical disruption' of lives by chronic illness and suffering and the existential despair of embodiment, Deleuze and Guattari's position offers the possibility for a subjectivity not limited by the body-with-organs. Meanings are capable of transformation, with possibilities for *deterritorialization*. Part of that process may be the dissolution of systems of thought deriving from biomedicine, mind–body dualism (which sees the mind as 'trapped' inside the body), and the interior–exterior conception of subjectivity. The individualizing of pain and suffering by biomedicine (often with the collaboration of the human sciences) territorializes an organism (a body-*with*-organs) upon the BwO: a body-with-organs which is then the natural subject for the expertise of medicine. I shall now consider this notion of *territorialization* (and the concomitant possibility of deterritorialization) in greater detail.

Territorialization

We need to see how everyone, at every age, in the smallest things as in the greatest challenges, seeks a territory, tolerates or carries out deterritorializations, and is reterritorialized on almost anything – memory, fetish or dream. (Deleuze and Guattari 1994: 67–8)

Deleuze and Guattari see territorialization (*deterritorialization* and *reterritorialization*) as the outcome of the dynamic relation between forces (physical and psychosocial) and apply this general conception to the specific arena of the ascription of meaning to the social relations of human life. Thus the act of taking a branch and turning it into a tool is both a material *and* a phenomenological reterritorialization. Concomitantly, a sharpened stick is a deterritorialized branch (Deleuze and Guattari 1994: 67). Under capitalism, the merchant deterritorializes products into commodities, while labour is abstracted, becoming reterritorialized as wages (ibid.: 68). Territories and deterritorializations can be not only physical but also psychological and spiritual: philosophy and ideology reterritorialize land as Homeland or Fatherland (ibid.). These systems of thought (what Foucault called 'discourses') possess authority, and as such may deterritorialize and reterritorialize how we think about the world and about ourselves.

Territorialization is an active process, whose agent may be human, animate, inanimate or abstracted (society, God, 'they'), as may the object of territorialization. Thus the force of the sun's gravity territorializes the earth in its travels through space, acting on it through the exertion of a force. Similarly, the air blown through a reed is territorialized to vibrate and produce a musical tone through the action of a musician's lungs. In the realm of the social, territorializations also occur through the action of forces. The first part of this book was concerned with a range of such forces, from the silencing of patients following surgery (chapter 1), the limitations of time and space (chapter 2) and the organization of care (chapter 3). Usually (though not always) these social territorializations entail – somewhere in the process – some act of interpretation, of ascribing meaning to an act or action.

The metaphor of territorialization is used to great effect in Chatwin's *The Songlines* (1987) in which he follows the paths of Australian aboriginal peoples across their land. Just as birds sing to mark their territory (Deleuze and Guattari 1988: 312), human songs can do the same. Chatwin describes how aboriginal people 'sing their world into existence' as they trace out the journeys which their totemic ancestors travelled across the land. The song – of the aboriginal person, or of a child in the dark or a person doing housework (Deleuze and Guattari 1988: 311) – territorializes the chaos which is the Universe, but in the process *deterritorializes* the BwO of the singer. The child is no longer afraid, the aboriginal person no longer lost, as the song ascribes *meaning* to the environment and to his or her relation with it.

Human beings (and dogs and crows) territorialize others and themselves as they act in ways sensible to them. For the dog and the crow, we might conceptualize sense as the accretion of behaviours proper to their species as they interact with the environment: the phenotypical manifestation of a genotype of potentiality. Human beings – at least, so we believe – are unique in their additional capacity for a reflexive sense-making through the mediation of language, and territorialization will not simply follow predisposition because of the undecidability of language.

The will-to-power of the human being is its capacity to act upon (territorialize) the world. But a territorialization of the other inevitably results in some reterritorialization of the BwO of the agent herself (the oppression of the victim makes the oppressor a tyrant, ministry to the sick sanctifies the healer). The will-to-power of the human being is thus (as Deleuze and Guattari call it), its *becoming* (1988: 277). Conversely, humans may become the subjects of deterritorialization and reterritorialization as the BwO is inscribed by the forces of the social: from birth (perhaps – one could argue – from conception) this inscription is a deterritorialization of virgin territory and a reterritorialization in some new patterning. The BwO is the summation of all these myriad deterritorializations and reterritorializations: it is in this sense that we might agree with Foucault's description of the body as totally imprinted by (its) history, but – I would add – *a history which has been enacted and engaged with, not simply imposed.*

Deleuze and Guattari identify the potential for resistance in this process of deterritorialization and reterritorialization, and of collective action to resist the forces of the social, as opposed to the individualized response of psychoanalysis to the territorialization of the psyche. They wish to be on the side of resistance, and argue that their work is in itself capable of deterritorializing the BwOs of its readers. At the outset of *A Thousand Plateaus* (a hypertextual book with chapters which are freestanding and may be read in any order), Deleuze and Guattari (1988: 6–7) argue that writing can be *rhizomatic*. The rhizome is subterranean and subversive, multiple and diverse in form, but more importantly

> has no beginning or end; it is always in the middle, between things, interbeing, *intermezzo*. ... The tree imposes the verb 'to be', but the fabric of the rhizome is the conjunction 'and ... and ... and ...'.
> (Deleuze and Guattari 1988: 25)

Similarly the actions of others as they impinge on a person can be rhizomatic, the line of flight (ibid.: 9) by which the BwO escapes from a territorialization. Often the deterritorialization is momentary and perhaps inconsequential: the BwO moves just a little from its previous position before reterritorializing in a new patterning. At other times, it may be substantial and life-changing, a line of flight which carries the BwO into unimagined realms of possibility and becoming-other. To give two examples: a patient's BwO may be deterritorialized by the health-care worker or friend who treats her as something more than a collection of pathologies; the child's BwO may be deterritorialized (and reterritorialized) by the adult who treats her as an equal. Such lines of flight can enable what Deleuze and Guattari describe as *nomadic subjectivity*.

The Nomadic Subject and Nomadology

> A nomad knows how to wait – he [sic] has infinite patience. (Deleuze and Guattari 1988: 381)

All deterritorializations carry the trace of the nomadic in them, but Deleuze and Guattari distinguish between relative and absolute deterritorialization (Deleuze and Guattari 1988: 55). Because the relation between a person and her environment is dynamic and challenging, movements of deterritorialization and reterritorialization inhere in the dynamics of existence, and this can be seen clearly in relation to sickness and mortality. A risk to health from some environmental factor leads to a change in behaviour; illness or impairment force a person to adapt and exploit unused potentialities: in each case there is relative deterritorialization of the BwO.

These relative deterritorializations, even if they are very rapid or very extreme, rarely result in an absolute line of flight, the absolute deterritorialization of the BwO which Deleuze and Guattari call nomadism. Yet absolute deterritorialization is in a sense the precursor or the condition of territorialization: it is only because the BwO has been territorialized that deterritorialization becomes relative (1988: 56). There is always therefore the trace of absolute deterritorialization, of nomadism – both in relative deterritorializations and in the inscribed BwO itself. (I consider this in greater detail in chapter 8.) Deleuze and Guattari use the metaphor of the *nomad* to exemplify absolute deterritorialization.

> If the nomad can be called the Deterritorialized par excellence, it is precisely because there is no reterritorialization *afterward* as with the migrant, or upon something else as with the sedentary (the sedentary's relation with the earth is mediatized [sic] by something else, a property regime, a State apparatus). With the nomad on the contrary, it is deterritorialization that constitutes the relation with the earth, to such a degree that the nomad reterritorializes on deterritorialization itself. (ibid.: 381, their emphasis)

The nomad follows customary paths, but only so that she may get from one point to the next; the points possess no significance other than this. They do not mark out territory to be distributed among people (as with sedentary cultures), rather people are distributed in an open space without borders or enclosures. Nomad space is smooth, without features, and in that sense the nomad traverses without movement, the land ceases to be other than support. Unlike the migrant, the nomad does not leave land because it has become hostile: she clings to the smoothness of the space she inhabits (ibid.: 380–1).

In a telling phrase, Deleuze and Guattari suggest that what is needed – in opposition to history – is nomadology (Deleuze and Guattari 1988: 23). History is written from the point of view of the sedentary, the State apparatus. Nomadology multiplies narratives, is an uninterrupted flow of deterritorialization which inhabits the smooth untextured space of existence without reterritorializing it into a single grand design. So nomadology must be thought of not as a state (and there are no nomads anyway, only nomadism) but as a process, as a line of flight which continually resists the sedentary, the single fixed perspective. Recalling that Foucault spoke of the body completely imprinted with history – that is, the forces of the social; the objective of nomadology is a *nomad subjectivity* free to roam on the surface of the BwO, untrammelled by the territorializations of power, free to *resist*.

Yet it is hard to be a nomad, especially when one has been sedentary, like a farmer with a relation to the land based on property, produce and productivity: few farmers leave their land willingly; to do so requires a change in perspective. Nomadic subjects, like Buddhists, aspire to shed attachment, to engage with the world without letting it possess one's soul. The line of flight which deterritorializes always tends toward a reterritorialization: one is only ever *becoming*-nomad.

The Politics of (Dis)embodiment

A body (*corps*) is not reducible to an *organism*, any more than esprit de corps is reducible to the soul of the organism. Spirit is not better, but it is volatile, whereas the soul is weighted, a centre of gravity. (Deleuze and Guattari 1988: 366, their emphases)

Having set out some of the fundamentals of Deleuze and Guattari's position, I want to apply these ideas to my project of rethinking health and illness. From what has gone before, it is clear that Deleuze and Guattari's project is political, and that nomadology represents a political commitment to resistance and to difference. In this politics both the nomadic subject and the terrain over which she passes are transformed from the relations of territorialization, which constitute subjects and their environments as territories to be inhabited, annexed, battled over.

Another way of thinking of this politics is as a politics of disembodiment, in the sense of the constructed Bodies-without-Organs which Deleuze and Guattari speak about. Just one of these embodiments is the *body-with-organs* of biomedicine and its acolytes, although this is a powerful version of the Body-without-Organs. Nomadology is the disembodiment, the divestment of embodiment, the unshackling of the full BwO, which as will be recalled, Deleuze and Guattari describe as 'unproductive, ... sterile, ... unengendered, ... unconsumable' (Deleuze and Guattari 1984: 8).

The politics of disembodiment cannot – of course – be the return to some prior status before the inscription of the BwO created subjectivity: that can be achieved only through annihilation. At best what can be achieved is a *plateau*, a space in which becoming-other is possible, if only for a moment (Massumi 1992: 7). So what precisely *is* entailed in this project of disembodiment, and how might it be applied? Because thinking about nomadology is itself part of the rhizomatic from which nomadic subjectivity emerges (Deleuze and Guattari 1988: 24), a rhizomic manoeuvre may be of use at this point. Through the convergences and divergences of other post-structuralist theory and in examples of practice, we may gain a clearer view of how we might act in this political realm.

Derrida, Meaning and the Frame

Deconstruction, the approach developed by Derrida (1976) to explore the workings of power in the textual construction of the social world, has been applied in social theory to reveal the unspoken assumptions behind claims to 'truth' (Fox 1991, 1993a, Game 1991). It is of particular use in exploring how particular systems of thought come to dominance, and what happens in situations where interpretations of reality are contested. In general, it works by overturning these privileged readings, examining the way the world would look if the opposing view were to be dominant. As such, it is potentially both anti-authoritarian and a tool for resistance (Critchley 1992, Rosenau 1992).

As was illustrated in chapter 1, part of Derrida's deconstructive analysis of how meaning is achieved (in other words how one reading comes to have sense for a reader) is through the *framing* of a text. Thus, Derrida described in *The Truth in Painting* how a picture establishes its subject-matter more from what it excludes from the canvas (including the painter herself) than from what is included. A poem chooses a few words to convey its message, but those words draw their power from the discipline of the form. It may be stylized as a *haiku* or a sonnet, or draw on techniques of assonance or tonality, *excluding* the more extended narrative of the novel or conversation. In studies of the social there are many examples of such delimiting acts. Thus, for instance, 'normality' is defined at its limits, at the points at which deviances begin; professions define themselves by excluding routine or unskilled labour.

Derrida argues that the authority which ascribes meaning to a text, and which in turn achieves the power to make such claims, acts at the frame, the limit or the margin. Indeed, without a frame, there is no authority. This understanding of how power establishes meaning is helpful in conceptualizing the BwO, and how its 'in-folding' of the social creates a subject. At the heart of Derrida's model is the engine (the manufacturer) of difference: language. Similarly, the model of the BwO is differential, the on-going patterning of intensities which establish a territory (Deleuze and Guattari 1988: 70). The BwO is inscribed by difference, by what differentiates it from what it is not: subjectivity is the outcome of a strategic limitation. Like any territory, it is meaningful because it is bounded and in relation to what is excluded from it, subjectivity becomes a conscious reflexivity only at the margins, limits and boundaries, just as property rights make sense only through determining boundaries.

Deterritorialization is the destruction of limits, of their rendition as no longer 'meaningful'. The politics of disembodiment must be aware of these limits, of how they create through their exclusions. Exposing a frame exposes the power which is at work in territorialization; once exposed, it can no longer frame because what is beyond has become part of what is enclosed. Deconstruction *is* deterritorialization. It follows that part of the project of destabilising power, authority and control will entail the meticulous unpicking of concepts, beliefs and assumptions, of questioning why things are the way they are, and suggesting how they might be different. The politics of such an enterprise is familiar territory for, amongst others, feminist theorists.

Cixous, Haraway and the Cyborg

It has been said that there are only two genres of autobiography, that of the hero and that of the dispossessed. Both genres exist in relation to territorialization. The hero has control of her territory, the dispossessed is defined by her exclusion from it. In this sense the BwO of the hero and of the dispossessed are equivalent, both are territorialized, but stand at the margin, though looking in opposite directions. 'Writing at the margins' (a terminology which has been applied to the writing of women, of black people, of others excluded from power in phallogocentric culture) can serve as a marker for that boundary. And, as was suggested in the previous section, once a boundary is exposed, its power begins to fail.

Intertextuality is the play of text on text, the inevitable process which is put in train as soon as a reader approaches a text (be it a written text, another symbolic medium or a social practice capable of interpretation). It is a feature of the undecidability of social interaction, of the multiplication of meaning which refuses a single territorialization. While all texts possess this 'semiotic' quality, texts which actively encourage multiplicity may be of particular value in the politics of disembodiment.

For a number of feminist post-structuralists including Julia Kristeva and Helene Cixous, writing has just this significance. Kristeva speaks of a 'poetic' which is not governed by the (masculine) symbolic rules of syntax but in the 'semiotic' (Kristeva 1986). This semiotic feminine principle is marginal, it plays guerrilla tactics with a text's meaning, though it is always doomed to fall back into the register of the symbolic as a fixity of meaning is established by a reader. This echoes Derrida's assertion of the undecidability of the text, but it also reminds us of the deterritorialization of meaning which Deleuze and Guattari describe.

Cixous's *écriture feminine* is a writing practice which is concerned with the openness of texts and multiplicity in place of closure and univocality (Game 1991: 80): feminine texts strive to undermine oppositions (margins), to deconstruct textuality itself, opening up the prison-house of patriarchal language (Moi 1985: 107). As was noted in chapter 3, for Cixous the masculine realm is that of the *proper* (associated with property, propriety, appropriation), opposed to the feminine realm of the *gift* based in generosity. Comparing these realms in the context of *écriture feminine*, Cixous writes that

> A feminine text cannot fail to be more than subversive. It is volcanic: as it is written it brings about an upheaval of the old property crust, carrier of masculine investments ... it's in order to smash everything, to shatter the framework of institutions, to blow up the law, to break up the 'truth' with laughter. (Cixous 1990: 326)

Cixous's analysis may be taken as simply advocating a writing practice which opens up possibilities for others (a *gift*) through a fragmentation of meaning, similar to Deleuze and Guattari's commendation of their book *A Thousand Plateaus* as a rhizome which can be employed as a tool of nomadology. However, Cixous's advocacy of *écriture feminine* as a political strategy may also be understood as based on an intertextuality between language and the female body, challenging the Cartesian dualism of mind/body and incorporating the body into signification (Banting 1992: 239). However, the relationship between body and language (concept, discourse, body of knowledge) is based not on representation but upon translation, in the way the hysteric's body is a translation between language and flesh, speaking eloquently where language fails to enunciate the oppression of being female (ibid.: 231, 240).

The body is poetic, a pictogram, full of meaning, yet irreducible to language. In this sense, the body is itself a form of 'writing': the *arché-writing* conceived by Derrida (1976: 56) as the system of differences or *différance* which makes language possible. *Ecriture feminine* becomes a means of deterritorialization of the BwO, acting on the side of nomad thought. Banting argues that

> Cixous does not restrict *écriture feminine* to translation between language and the body. She invites us to translate from the patriarchal vernaculars towards languages more amenable to women and others and to let such acts of translation work to re-inscribe and re-organise our bodies. (1992: 240)

Whether or not there is an essentialism in Cixous's work (Moi (1985) argues aye, Banting (1992) nay to this proposition), her conception of *écriture feminine* as a form of resistance has a congruence which the other perspectives developed in this chapter. It suggests the active involvement of the Body-without-Organs in territorialization and deterritorialization, that the body is a site both of inscription and resistance.

Donna Haraway describes her tale of cyborgs as a myth (1991: 154), and we can see in this myth features of Cixous's *écriture feminine*: a story which challenges boundaries and opens up new ways of thinking ourselves. While in traditional science and politics (and I might add, sociology), human and machine (nature and culture) are at odds, her story is '… an argument for *pleasure* in the confusion of boundaries and *responsibility* in their construction' (ibid.: 150). Like the woman, created at the margin, the cyborg is a chimera:

> The cyborg is resolutely committed to partiality, irony, intimacy and perversity. It is oppositional, utopian, and completely without inno-cence. … Nature and culture are reworked; the one can no longer be the resource for appropriation or incorporation by the other. … The cyborg would not recognise the Garden of Eden; it is not made of mud and cannot dream of returning to dust. … They are wary of holism, but

needy for connection – they seem to have a natural feel for united front politics, but without the vanguard party. (ibid.: 151)

The cyborg myth, she goes on, is about transgressed boundaries, potent fusions and dangerous possibilities which can be explored as part of a progressive politics which rejects dualisms in an effort to seek new meanings and forms of power and pleasure (ibid.: 154). Thinking a chimera dissolves old prejudices and makes conscious old repressions. In other words, it deterritorializes, while proffering new territory for invest-ment. Of course, a deterritorialization is often followed by a reterritorialization of the BwO, and cyborgs are not *per se* on the side of resistance: Haraway argues that the (post)modern world is filled with cyborgs, and that it is their ubiquity and invisibility which makes them such powerful political tools, for repression as well as for resistance (ibid.: 153–4).

So the cyborg, the transgressor of boundaries, is a further tool for a politics of disembodiment, challenging and questioning the territorializa-tions of science, biomedicine, the law and religion. Recall my descriptions of the cyborgs Stellarc and Orlan in the introductory chapter: their exper-iments with the limits of the body challenge and undermine body boundaries and norms, testing the limits of what it is to be 'human'. The debates over the medical fusions of human and machine: from the hip replacement to the cloned sheep, from genetically engineered plants and animals to virtual reality sexual encounters are like Cixous's volcanic texts; they smash all before them as they challenge boundaries and disturb safe and comfortable dualities.

From role-playing and fantasy games to gender-bending and computer-mediated interactions in MUDs and MOOs (virtual spaces enabling non-corporeal interactions), information and communication technolo-gies enable nomadic subjectivities to emerge, freed from the constraints of human limits or physical embodiment (Rushkoff 1994). Yet these latter engagements remind us how easy it is to slip into territorialization. The imaginativeness of the interactions which occur in such environments are often depressingly limited, caught up in narrow notions of the erotic and the possible, and often harking back to a territorialization based in the familiar territories of 'reality' (Fox and Roberts 1999, Stone 1992).

The cyborg is not necessarily a nomad, but perhaps has reached a 'plateau', to use Deleuze and Guattari's term, in which there are new possi-bilities to be explored and enjoyed. Becoming-cyborg is maybe a step towards nomadology.

Lines of Flight: Growing Older or Just Growing?

I want to bring the lines of flight which have developed in the course of this chapter – if not exactly down to earth, at least to fully engage with the theme of this book. I will once again do this in relation to some of my work on care and how it is experienced. Specifically, I want to consider how the anti-essentialism of Deleuze and Guattari helps us to understand living and selfhood as a flux: a process of continual territorialization and deterritorialization, of constraint and resistance, of plateaus and nomadism.

Growing older might be reduced to the material effects of the passage of time on cells and organs. Yet, as we saw in chapter 2, we cannot make assumptions about time and what it does to bodies. Physiologists agree that ageing is not an absolute: biological age does not equate to chronological age. Even if we accept that cells age, that life on the surface of this planet changes and often degrades human tissue, we cannot reduce the experience of being 'old' to the biological. At the simplest level, when I interviewed 'old' people in Thailand that meant people over 60, while old Australians were 65 or more: that was how these different cultures defined being old.

So what was the BwO of the older adult in my study like? The answer to that is: they were as diverse as the people themselves. For many of the Thai respondents, a major territorialization affecting the experience of becoming older was associated with Buddhist beliefs.

Thai Mr A: My daughter would take care of me, but I don't need it at present. I would like to help myself, and because I am a Buddhist, I want to obtain peace by using the middle way. I would like just to stay by myself. ... If my daughter can stay with me I will be very happy, but I haven't asked her to take care of me. I am trying to understand how to use the Buddha, if someone concentrates on religion they can understand and this makes me happy. After meditation I feel very light in my body, and very light in my mind.

Thai Mr O: It is a good thing to be an old person, I feel good if there is someone to take care of me, and my body will go to the hospital after I die. It is a good way to live, I don't worry about his life or about anything. It is the Buddhist philosophy: don't worry about anything, don't worry about your body, your life in the long run, I will give everything in the long run to the Government. ... Religion is very important to me, to give respect to the Buddha, and do meditation every day. I am a very strict Buddhist.

For the Australians, there was no such overarching philosophy or world-view to bolster a sense of their humanity. Fatalism and a general stoicism seemed to structure how some of the older adults thought about their life.

Australian Mrs S: I don't think about the future very much. We've just got to live a quiet life and we know quite a few of the people around. There are different things we can do. We can read although I'm getting to the stage where I can't read, and that's a bit of a disappointment because I thought I would always be able to read. I think I live quite a dull life now, but the family are good.

Australian Mrs K: I think it's all right. I don't mind it. You've all got to get old. You can't avoid it.
Mr K: If you're lucky. You see, when you're 40, you're 40 per cent in the grave and after that it becomes 50, 60, 70 and 100, doesn't it? You don't realize that – at 60 years of age, you're 60 per cent dead. You've only got 40 per cent left. What you do with that 40 per cent is up to you.

Becoming dependent on others – financially, physically or emotionally – might be experienced either as a positive aspect of growing older, or as something which reduced the older persons' capacity to see themselves as in control of their lives. Most of the Thai respondents found positive aspects to this sense of dependency, indeed they sometimes found it hard to grasp that this was anything other than the way things are naturally.

Karen (hill tribe) Mr H: Even if I am sick in my house, my son and daughter buy some tablets or medicine from the health centre or the chemist, or the grocery shop. ... I am sure my son will stay with me, because when he gets married, he will bring his wife to stay with him.
NF (via interpreter): When he was younger, he looked after his children. Now they look after him. Does that seem strange to him?
Mr H: No, I don't feel strange, this is the way of life – we look after them when they are children, and now I am old they have to look after me. This is our lifestyle ... because their duty ... even my daughter got married and lives not far from here, they quite often ask about my eating, or my health ...

Thai Mrs G: I'm not dependent on my children, because I help myself with the things that I can do. My children give me some food, take care of me, but I help myself first. I can walk, I can do anything. It is the good Buddhist philosophy, that I helped my mother, and my children take care of me. ... People should do the good thing, so they receive the good thing back. If they don't do good things, they will receive bad things back.

Once again, the Australian older adults had a less territorialized sense of themselves in relation to others, but dependency weighed heavily as it increased the territorialization of their lives and selves. The sense of autonomy, of having a 'nomadic subjectivity' was removed: a painful process.

Australian Mrs C: You feel as if everything's taken from you. That's what it seems like and it's very hard to accept. But anyhow I've got used to it now. You've lost your independence. You've lost things. And you've got to rely on these people. And that's all about it. You've got to just settle down and get used to it, and that's it. Which I have in no time flat; I just had to and make a damn good job. No good saying, 'I don't want to' because there's nothing else you can do.

Australian Mrs A: ... you lose your responsibility when you come into these sort of places and you haven't got that, you know, to be responsible for – the shopping, the cleaning, the cooking and everything. When you come in here, you haven't got that responsibility and it's not good to have no responsibility for anything. And that is very hard.

This reterritorialization was reflected in various ways, as the social impinged differently for each individual. For some, economic and physical reliance on others meant a loss of autonomy. For one older Thai man, the struggle to get enough to eat was exacerbated by his co-residence with his son's family.

Thai Mr P: I would prefer to stay on my own, or if I could be just with my son it would be OK, but it's my daughter-in-law, if I buy something to eat then everybody eats my food! Old people should be with their family, but my son has so many people in the house. My son pays all the expenses and takes care of me. Yesterday he took me to the hospital because I had asthma. But I am lonely and do not get enough to eat. Every day I watch the TV and read the newspaper.

This dependence on others, coupled with an economic downturn, territorialized some of the Australians living in hostel accommodation into a fearful BwO.

Australian Mr L: This government has cut funding enormously for a lot of older people. A lot of the people are frightened about what's going to happen, they don't know whether they'll be kept in here, whether they'll be thrown out or what. You don't expect that as you get older.
Mrs L: If we get thrown out of here, we've got nowhere to go. We've sold our unit and we've sold our home.
Mr L: When we first came here, we had enough that we could go out and have a dinner at a hotel. Now, we just haven't got enough money. It means we have to stay in here.

For many of the respondents, the negative side of growing older was clearly associated with infirmity, and the loss of capacities to act as they had done when younger. 'Keeping your health' was crucial, and it was perceived as something which had been 'taken away' as a result of getting older. But health or lack of it was not in itself what was sought or feared. Rather in the way that time (as we saw in chapter 2) was a commodity which could buy or be bartered for desired commodities or states, 'health' was something which enabled, and its loss was blamed for the reterritorialization which old age brought.

Australian Mrs C: You think about old times, that's when you ask 'Why should it be me?' People at my age are still going like anything and I can't, that's what gets me down. You see people of 80 getting round, good as gold, not me. I've just got to put up with what I've got. If I could get around more, I wouldn't be here, not yet. The doctor reckons it's hereditary. My dad died of a heart attack; my brother had an operation on the heart; my sister's had an operation. ... I live from day to day now.

Hmong (hill tribe) Mrs J: For old people it's not good because sometimes, quite often, they are sick and have no energy to go in the fields or the mountains. I go to work in the field four days per week, or if I don't go to the field, I get up early to cook, after that sewing, and after that I cook dinner and go to bed. Sometimes I feel unhappy because my children have grown up, some of them go out to work in the field, or have gone to study in the city. I feel lonely.

Even when in relatively good physical fitness, the fear of future infirmity was sometimes a factor territorializing how the respondents thought about ageing.

Thai Mrs Q: I don't like being an old person, because old people have many problems about health. If old people are healthy it is OK, it is good to be an old person. I can do many activities, like go out to the temple for many recreations. ... I would like health education, to give information on how to eat good food although sometimes I can't afford good food.

Australian Mr L: If you've got your health I guess it makes a difference. When I first came here I used to have a vegetable garden growing down the side there. Emphysema gets progressively worse and there's nothing they can do for you. Well, I can't do the garden now so I've lost that interest. I would like to get involved in some of the other activities, like bowling, but I can't do that because I can't bend down. I just think it would be different if you got old and you'd got your health. If your health goes, your spirit's gone and I think that's the thing.

This data suggests that for many people I spoke with, becoming older was a territorializing experience. Security and basic welfare, health and activity, and more existential concerns with autonomy and selfhood, all contributed to a territorialization of the BwOs, in ways contextual to their lives and cultures. Yet there was no 'loss of self' among these older adults. They were not flickering candles being extinguished by the cold draughts of privation. Rather, they were engaged and motivated people, resisting and refusing the limits – the territorializations – which ageing, infirmity and institutionalization imposed.

But could growing older also be a *deterritorialization*? In chapter 3, I documented some of the positive comments from the Australians living in residential accommodation about the pleasure of being cared for by committed and loving staff. Both in Thailand and Australia, many of the people I spoke to were very positive about aspects of being older, of being cared for, and of having fewer responsibilities. Perhaps for them, the character of relationships had changed, from the reciprocity of youth, to an acceptance of being a recipient. Unable to give anything back, they had somehow become more fulfilled in themselves.

Thai Mrs L: I don't think about being old, in my mind I am still a school child because here we have everything, we have many activities. Where I live, it's just like a child who came to school. In the morning I come to the front of this home, and sing the national song, and at eight o'clock I go to the cafeteria here and at nine p.m. I go to bed. ... I feel good because the caregiver will take care of me, and a lot of people come to visit us and take care, and make some activities for us. I used to think that the people in these homes were people the family doesn't want, and let them come here. But now I don't think that, because the elderly people are more important and a lot of people outside see the importance of the elderly and come to visit me, make activities that entertain me.

Australian Mr W: When I'm out walking, I can't see, but I always say good morning, and they always respond. And even the school kids, they will say good morning, you know. And that gives you a sort of a warm glow when kids are wishing you good morning.

For these older adults, age had brought all sorts of changes, not only in material life, but significantly, in how they understood themselves and their lives and biographies. Chronological age and the passage of time, economic and physical dependency, fear about the future, infirmity or incapacity: all were factors in reterritorializing the BwOs of older adults. It is not that they were not previously free of territorialization. Personal biographies, material circumstances, embodiment and culture all had made them what they were, had been contingencies as they 'made' their Bodies-without-Organs (Deleuze and Guattari 1988: 149) from their moment of conception.

Nor was it the case that the changes which age brought were absolutes. Some of the Thai people I met lived in economic and material conditions which would have been insupportable for a westerner, while the relative luxury of the residential homes in Australia would have been unimaginable for many Thai folk. Similarly, the lens of culture changed how age was to be understood: its relevance for how people saw themselves in relation to the cosmos, and the meaning of their lives.

So there is not a simple 'hierarchy of needs' (Maslow 1968) here, with security and material provision fundamental for the 'higher' needs of autonomy and self-realization to be achieved. Sometimes, economic uncertainty could be the most territorializing aspect of growing older. For others, infirmity and the loss of freedom to do the simplest of activities were the most significant. On the other hand, even in the face of onto-logical challenges associated with death and impairment, some – notably the Buddhist Thais – found meaning and peace in the different phases of the life course. As one Thai said to me, 'it is good to be young, but it is also good to be old'.

So nomadology must engage with material conditions as well as with the meanings which people ascribe to themselves and their situations. Yet it is also about how we move through our lives, to what we attach and from that which we detach. The value of Deleuze and Guattari's analysis is that both kinds of territorialization can be acknowledged by the perspective, and we can see an equivalence between the material circumstance and the meaning it has for one person or another. Both the change in a cell and the joy of seeing a sunset can be recognized as playing a part in making us who we are.

A Manifesto for Nomadism

In conclusion, I believe that there are three points which make Deleuze and Guattari's model important, and valuable for the project of moving beyond health.

First, that the body upon which the social world impinges is not the physical body. In the light of the previous chapter, readers will be aware that Foucault spoke of bodies disciplined and made passive by the authoritative systems of knowledge he called discourses. Prisoners, patients, workers were the objects of regimes of power focused on their bodies, and hence on their minds and souls (Foucault 1976: 89). A close reading of Foucault (for example 1977c: 169–70) suggests that the body he saw as disciplined was not physical, but something akin to the BwO of Deleuze and Guattari (Lash 1991: 264), a philosophical or psychic surface which could be inscribed with these discursive elements. The use of the term *Body-without-Organs* makes it clearer that the 'in-folding' of the social operates in a realm distant from the physical body, indeed that the sense we have of a physical body is a result of this patterning of the BwO.

Second, that the process of inscribing subjectivity is not a passive process, but a dynamic 'reading' of the social by an active, sense-making and motivated human being. For Deleuze and Guattari, the BwO is like an uncharted territory, but one whose possession must be fought over, inch by inch. Unlike Foucault's passive body, slowly but surely inscribed by civilization, for Deleuze and Guattari the BwO is always in flux, as it is territorialized, deterritorialized and reterritorialized endlessly. Territorialization is a function both of the forces of the social and by an opposing force, the 'affirmation of potential' which is the will-to-power of the human, which might be understood as the motivated and engaged sense-making of the BwO as it becomes other. Thus the discourse of biomedicine is not passively inscribed on to the BwO, creating an image of itself. Rather the territorialization is resisted and subverted, so that what ends up being inscribed is in no sense a simulacrum, but a patterning which may bear some, or perhaps only a slight, resemblance to the territorializing force.

And what is inscribed may be deterritorialized by other forces of the social, or as other forces of deterritorialization impinge. What is offered here is a dynamic model, one which can conjure the endless permutations of the social, and which is intertextual: the result of a myriad of texts written one over the other. The BwO is the ultimate reader, always capable of a new interpretation, another nuance.

Third, because the process of territorialization of the BwO is dialogical, there is the possibility for resistance. The inscription of the BwO is not monolithic, but occurs in dynamic tension with conflicting forces. Just as physical forces may be marshalled to produce a vector whose direction is that of none of the individual forces, the patterns of intensity which inscribe the BwO can supply unexpected directions for subjectivity: lines of flight which can break a subject free to wander like a nomad for a while, before settling back in a new and unprecedented configuration or reterritorialization (Massumi 1992: 7–8). Resistance is not only a possibility, it is the character of the BwO. The politics of disembodiment is about engaging with the real struggles of people as they are territorialized, as they resist, and as they encourage others in the aspiration to nomadic subjectivity.

These conclusions provide the basis for a non-essentialist understanding of a resisting subject. In the final part of the book, this model will be used to address the political project of nomadic embodiment beyond health.

Part 3
BECOMING

Introduction

The trouble with resistance is that – unless one keeps doing it – either the force which had motivated the resistance reasserts itself, or what had been the objective for which the act of resistance was constituted, becomes the new orthodoxy. The history of the past two centuries Is replete with examples of the latter. The socialist revolution to resist capitalism becomes the establishment of the communist state; the Islamic rebellion in Iran to depose the despot introduces oppression no less aggressive, if differently focused. The white racism of colonialism is replaced with a tribal hegemony which leads to genocide and a new rule of force. No turning away of this kind is absolute, once and for all (Deleuze and Guattari 1994: 96); there is always a moment at which resistance seems to have delivered the goods, and with the relaxation of effort, force is reasserted – one way or another.

So is it easier to stop resisting, to acknowledge force as a fact of life and give in? Conducting all-out war, or even a guerrilla campaign, becomes wearing after years of struggle. Look at what happened to the women's movement or the trade unions: they called it a day and now we have post-feminism and New Labour! Refusing and resisting is too much like hard work; let's settle for what we've got: after all we've dented patriarchy and capitalism, given them a make-over.

In the final section of this book, having developed a theory of a non-essential resisting subject which holds up, we have to ask the question: why bother? If resistance is ultimately futile, either acquiescing to force or reintroducing a new order of force, what's the point of it all? In the context of the subject of this book: embodiment and 'health', why not settle for the inevitable in the face of the forces of modern discipline? Why struggle for an alternative which will be just as constraining qualitatively?

I want to use the remainder of the book to argue that resistance is not futile, but that it can be transformed from a negative into a positive. Once again the figure I shall invoke is the *nomad* – who wanders, but not aimlessly (which is why Bauman's (1993a) alternative icon: the *vagabond* – who is simply a bum – won't do) from place to place, taking what is useful and leaving behind what cannot be applied fruitfully at that point. A nomadic subjectivity is a resisting subjectivity, but one which does not simply refuse, but acts positively, meeting force with force to create a new vector, a new *line of flight*.

The line of flight is the way beyond, and cultivating such lines is crucial for the project of *becoming-other* about which I will have much to say in the coming pages. I shall show how we need to understand the body and embodiment processually, rather than thinking of the body as a thing or an entity with fixed properties and characteristics. Each chapter is itself a line of flight, disrupting and overturning, but productively rather than with destructive consequences. In these three chapters I do not even attempt to address every aspect of living: as if I knew all the answers – there are no answers anyway, only good questions. But I plan to *evoke* (Tyler 1986) the mood of the nomad as well as *analysing* her qualities. Each chapter is designed to stand alone: to speak one of myriad truths, to fracture force and promote becoming.

Chapter 6 selects a topic which goes to the heart of embodiment, the burgeoning literature and 'ethics of existence' on risky behaviour and safe behaviour. According to some writers, we now live in a 'risk society' (Beck 1994) in which we must be vigilant about the proliferation of risks. We must behave accordingly, limiting our actions to avoid these risky situations. The consequence: a subjectivity which is trammelled by fear and restricted by the prognostications of the risk analyst. I pull apart the arguments about risk, to suggest that risk analysis is not neutral, but is based on a privileged view of how human beings should act. Using two areas – health at work and the use of street drugs – I argue that it is possible to resist and refuse the risk analysts and choose actions which enhance and open up possibilities.

Research is at the heart of risk analysis, and in chapter 7 I focus on the practice of research, challenging the modernist perspective that there is a truth out there to be discovered. Instead, I suggest there are 'truths' which are setting contingent. I offer two models for a postmodern or nomadic research process: a focus on reflexivity and an exploration of action research. The latter challenges researcher/researched dichotomies and leads to an engaged and transgressive approach to knowledge and understanding.

The final chapter dives back into Deleuze and Guattari's work for a final exercise in grasping nomadology and what it means for embodiment. I argue that embodiment must be seen as an unfinished project. Two themes emerge in these final pages: a commitment to resistance and an ethico-political orientation towards engagement with the world (rather than a detachment and individualistic attitude). I make some suggestions for the practice of nomadology, and end with a short reflection on what the nomadic perspective has meant for me.

6
Risks and Choices

Having established the basis for thinking about a subjectivity which – while not essential – is capable of resistance, I want to look further at the ways in which notions of 'health' territorialize subjects, and what it might mean to challenge that territorialization. Rather than focus on aspects of hospitalization or care as in the first part of this book, I shall consider here a key element of how health has been thought of over the past decade, and to which social sciences have made a major contribution. This is the area of health behaviour, particularly in relation to 'risk'. Two areas of 'risky behaviour' will be considered: workplace hazards associated with blood products, and the use of street drugs such as Ecstasy. I will argue for a re-evaluation of the languages of risk, to suggest a new emphasis on choice and possibility.

Before the era of modernity, *risk* was a neutral term, concerned merely with probabilities, of losses and gains. A gamble or an endeavour that was associated with high risk meant simply that there was great potential for significant loss or significant reward. However, in the modern period, *risk* has been co-opted as a term reserved for a negative or undesirable outcome, and as such is synonymous with the terms *danger* or *hazard*. Thus the British Medical Association's guide *Living with Risk* describes a *hazard* as 'a set of circumstances which may cause harmful consequences', while *risk* is 'the likelihood of its doing so' (1987: 13). Furthermore, this hazard/risk differentiation introduces a moral dimension, such that the perpetrators of *risk* may be held to account in some way or other (Douglas 1992: 22–5). This chapter explores this dichotomy, and develops a postmodern position that challenges more traditional readings.

The science of risk calculation, assessment and evaluation is emblematic of modernism and its commitments to progress through rationalization: from the actuarial tables of life insurers to the risk analysis of those in the business of risk: the movers and shakers of capitalism (Hassler 1993). In what might almost be a handbook for such entrepreneurial activity, Johnstone-Bryden, in a monograph sub-titled *How to Work Successfully with Risk,* offers a blueprint for 'how risks can be identified and reduced economically and effectively, before serious damage occurs' (1995: 1). Hertz and Thomas (1983: 1) describe risk analysis as methods which seek a 'comprehensive understanding and awareness' of the risks associated with a given setting.

Risk assessment, we are led to believe by such authors, is a technical procedure which, like all aspects of modern life, is to be undertaken through rational calculation of ends and means (Fox 1991). Figure 6.1, based on an illustration of the process of risk assessment in a UK government publication, suggests the 'simple, logical sequence of steps' (Department of the Environment 1995: 5) to be taken to identify and manage risk. This process of risk assessment has been widely applied to many areas of technology over the past half century (Carter 1995: 135). Within such a scenario, all risks may be evaluated and suitably managed, such that all may be predicted and countered, so risks, accidents and insecurities are minimized or prevented altogether (Johnstone-Bryden 1995: 3, Prior 1995).

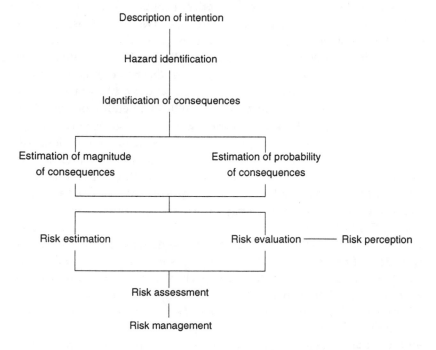

Figure 6.1 From intention to risk management

Such accounts fail to problematize risk and its assessment, and a range of social science analyses have been developed to offer a more critical approach, which address the socially constructed and historically specific character of such conceptualization of risk and its assessment. At the simplest level, we may conclude that 'risk is in the eye of the beholder':

> Insurance experts (involuntarily) contradict safety engineers. While the latter diagnose zero risk, the former decide: uninsurable. Experts are undercut or deposed by opposing experts. Politicians encounter the resistance of citizens' groups, and industrial management encounters morally and politically motivated consumer boycotts. (Beck 1994: 11)

In Beck's typification of contemporary western civilization as a 'risk society' (Beck 1992, 1994), the proliferation of risks as a consequence of technological innovation has got out of control. The success of modernist instrumental rationality has led to an apparent solution through technology to every problem, ill or need. But alongside the development of technology, and – for those who may earn a living through such innovation – the accumulation of wealth, Beck suggests there is a concomitant accumulation of risks in undesirable abundance as a consequence of working with or consuming technology (1992: 22, 26). But, Beck goes on, risks

> only exist in terms of the (scientific or anti-scientific) *knowledge* about them. They can be changed, magnified, dramatised or minimised within knowledge, and to that extent they are particularly *open to social definition and construction.* (1992: 23, original emphases)

Furthermore, some people are more affected by the distribution and growth of risks, and there are winners and losers in risk definitions. Power and access to and control of knowledge thus become paramount in a risk society. This is the issue of *reflexivity* to which Beck alludes: society becomes a problem for itself (Beck 1994: 8).

> In risk issues, no one is an expert, or everyone is an expert, because all the experts presume what they are supposed to make possible and produce: cultural acceptance. The Germans see the world perishing along with their forests. The Britons are shocked by their toxic breakfast eggs: this is where and how their ecological conversion starts. (ibid.: 9)

This, for Beck, is a crisis for society in the late modern period, an opportunity for social critique, and ultimately a new emancipation coming in the wake

of the failure of socialism to provide a resolution to the inequities of capitalism (ibid.: 12). Reflexivity challenges the old status barriers of class and
control of wealth, creating new possibilities for coalition and organization.

In contrast to this kind of approach, and at the 'cultural' end of the
spectrum of social theories of risk, the work of anthropologist Mary
Douglas has been influential. In the same way she had explored the apparently irrational behaviour of both 'primitive' and 'civilized' peoples
(Douglas 1966) concerning fears over pollution, she identified

> the baffling behaviour of the public, in refusing to buy floodplain
> or earthquake insurance, in crossing dangerous roads, driving non-
> road-worthy vehicles, buying accident-provoking gadgets for the
> home, and not listening to the education on risks, all that continues
> as before. (Douglas 1992: 11)

Douglas suggested that the reason such behaviour seems baffling is the
failure to take culture into account. Using the typology of cultures developed
by herself and Aaron Widavsky (Douglas 1996) based on the two dimensions
of *grid* and *group* (reflecting degrees of social stratification and social solidarity respectively), she sought to illustrate how the risks one focused upon
as an individual had less to do with individual psychology (the discipline
informing rational choice theory and the health belief model) and more to
do with the social forms in which those individuals construct their understanding of the world and themselves (Douglas 1992:12). Further,

> If the cultural processes by which certain societies select certain kinds
> of dangers for attention are based on institutional procedures for allo-
> cating responsibility, for self-justification, or for calling others to
> account, it follows that public moral judgements will advertise certain
> risks powerfully, while the well-advertised risk will turn out to be
> connected with legitimating moral principles. (Rayner 1992: 92)

Three of the four possible combinations of high and low grid and group
are identified by Douglas in her most recent work (and developed and
explored in Rayner 1992) as cultural backcloths to risk decisions and
perceptions (the fourth – high grid/low group – comprises isolated, alien-
ated individuals). Douglas suggests that the remaining three combinations
can be seen in aspects of (late) modern culture. The low grid/low group
culture is typical of the competitive environment of the entrepreneurial
capitalist free market, in which individuals are untrammelled by restrictive
practices or rules. Also found in capitalist institutions are the high

grid/high group cultures where Weber's 'iron cage' of bureaucracy has regulated and incorporated systems and structures for interaction. The third kind of culture, low grid/high group are collectivist, egalitarian groups, which Douglas and others have suggested are found in voluntary groups including the anti-nuclear movement and political and religious cults (Douglas 1992: 77, Rayner 1992: 89).

What is considered as a risk, and how serious that risk is thought to be, will be perceived differently depending upon the organization or grouping to which a person belongs or identifies, as will the disasters, accidents or other negative occurrences which occur in a culture (Douglas 1992: 78). The free-market environment (low grid and low group) will see competitors as the main risk, to be countered by good teamwork and leadership. In the bureaucratic culture (high grid and high group), the external environment is perceived as generally punitive, and group commitment is the main way to reduce risk. Finally, in the voluntary culture (low grid with high group), the risks come from external conspiracies, and group members may be suspected of treachery.

This typology has been developed and related to empirical examples. Thus, for example, Douglas (1992: 102–21) explores the impact of these cultural dimensions of stratification and solidarity upon individual health responses to HIV contagion. The emphasis in this culturalist model of risk perception upon the *social* construction of risk is highly relevant for the explorations that follow.

Three Models of the Risk/Hazard Opposition

At the beginning of this chapter, I remarked upon the etymological constructions of *risk* and *hazard* in modernist discourse. Having explored the different positions of realist and culturalist analysts (as exemplified by Beck and Douglas), I now want to look at this in somewhat greater depth to consider the differing perspectives that are possible concerning the ontological relation of a *risk* to a *hazard*. While there is potential overlap between perspectives, for heuristic purposes I shall consider three possibilities, the last of which being what I shall call the *postmodern* position, with its emphasis on the textual fabrication of reality. I shall use two realms as exemplars of the differing positions: discussions of risks associated with the workplace and with street drug use.

Position 1: A risk maps directly on to an underlying hazard

The first position may be called realist or materialist, given the underlying ontology of a hazard as real and material. This is the perspective identified

at the beginning of the chapter, as the mapping of a *risk* (that is, the likelihood of an unpleasant occurrence) on to a *hazard* (the circumstances that
could lead to the occurrence). Thus the risks for health workers of
contracting hepatitis or other blood-related diseases are directly related
(amongst other things) to the hazard of working with sharps (hypodermic
needles etc.). The risk of side-effects from using street drugs derives from
the pharmacological properties of these drugs. Given the existence of
sharps in the work environment of a hospital nurse or doctor, or the pharmacological properties of drugs, there are associated probabilities of
negative outcomes from working in such environments or using illegal
drugs.

This is the position that is generally adopted in risk management and
assessment literature, where the objective is risk reduction (for example
Wells 1996: 6, van Leeuwen 1995: 3). Wells (1996: 1) describes a hazard as
something which 'has the potential to cause harm'. Given the presence of
the hazard, then strategies are to be adopted to minimize the likelihood
(the risk) that the hazard will be manifested in an unpleasant outcome.
The emphasis may be on individual education, individual or population
prevention measures or corporate strategy. As such, the position is not
inherently political, and may be co-opted to serve any or all of the
different interests which may engage discursively with the perceived
hazard, although often emphasizing an individualized approach to risk
analysis. Thus, Johnstone-Bryden suggests that

> People represent the real risk. Human greed, malice and error are the
> primary threats. It could be argued that almost every risk, perhaps even
> every risk, relates back to human error, or deliberate human actions.
> (1995: 57)

While the realist or materialist position may acknowledge that the level
of risk offered by a hazard is based on subjective judgement (Anand 1993),
the one-to-one mapping of risk on to hazard means that, while

> at no time will all of us agree on a single level of acceptable risk ... if
> people can agree upon the way risks are measured, and on the relevance
> of the levels of risk thus represented to the choices we must all make,
> then the scope for disagreement and dissent is thereby limited. (British
> Medical Association 1987: vii)

Despite the different value perspectives of analysts (for example, from
management, trade unions or pressure groups), the realist position estab-

lishes the potential for a formal process of scientific analysis of risks. I would suggest that such a claimed consensus over *how* to assess risk also creates the basis for moral judgements concerning implementation of risk reduction procedures, and implicitly, a culture of blame (although, as Douglas's typology implies, who is blamed may depend on who is the analyst).

Position 2: Hazards are natural, risks are cultural

In the second position, which might be called culturalist or constructionist, risks are opposed to hazards in the sense that while the latter are 'natural' and neutral, risks are the value-laden judgements of human beings concerning these natural events or possibilities. Within social science, this approach to risk has become more prominent. To focus again on Mary Douglas, despite her culturalist analysis which seeks to demonstrate that risks are perceived in a social context, she is keen to note that

> The dangers are only too horribly real ... this argument is not about the reality of the dangers, but about how they are politicised. ... Starvation, blight and famine are perennial threats. It is a bad joke to take this analysis as hinting that the dangers are imaginary. (Douglas 1992: 29)

This position has been the basis for a corpus of sociological analyses of risk perception. Two main themes emerge, first concerning the differing types of 'knowledge' which inform perceptions of risk, and second, the moral dimension to risk and risk-taking.

Concerning the constructed nature of 'knowledge', Thorogood (1995) surveyed patients' reflections on an imagined scenario of attending an HIV-positive dentist. She found patients keen to rely upon the professionalism of the dentist, not only to tell them if they were positive for the disease, but also because it was the dentist who possessed the professional knowledge of the risks involved. In return, they judged themselves responsible for reporting to their dentist if they – the patients – were HIV-positive.

Thorogood's study also illustrates the moral character of such judgements. Her respondents made such remarks as '... he wears gloves, uses a mask and a sterilizing unit, all you would expect from a good dentist' or '... he is a particularly nice dentist, everything is covered up': the moral qualities of the dentist are indicative of her or his hazardousness. Rogers and Salvage (1988: 106) report the other side of the coin, when they describe the stigmatizing by her manager of a nurse who had received a needlestick injury, and was required to use a marked cup, saucer and plate, even prior to a test result for HIV. Failure to abide by societal norms or rules may lead to victim-blaming. As Carter argues:

> those groups facing danger which can be defined as 'other' often face controls which work in the interests of the powerful 'same'. Thus a range of social practices exist, connected with risk assessment, which historically have often targeted specific groups ... the effect is to push the group into a space of danger – the place of the 'other'. Here they become a useful repository for our cultural ideas of danger. As long as we are 'good' ... then danger is elsewhere. (1995: 142–3)

Once again, such analyses can incline towards an individualization of risk assessment, and victim-blaming is particularly rife concerning aspects of life deemed societally deviant: for example, in the arenas of sexual behaviour and drug use. This moral dimension to risk assessment affects the allocation of resources within society to reduce the risks of various hazards. Risk reduction has costs attached to it – for society, for government, for industry or for individuals – and judgements must be made about the relative balance between costs and benefits (CCTA 1994: 16). From the culturalist perspective what is required is a sociologically-informed risk assessment, which can overcome the 'naiveté' of the technical scientific evaluation, and take into account the 'real world' of hazards, and how they impinge on the daily working lives of employees. Unfortunately, such a conclusion depends upon discovering an Archimedean spot outside of culture upon which to stand, and such spots are notoriously hard to find!

Position 3: Risk perceptions fabricate hazards

In addition to these two readings of the risk/hazard relationship, a third position is possible: the one which I shall call postmodern, and which I wish to explore in this chapter. It moves beyond the culturalist or constructionist model, to argue radically that hazards are *themselves* socially constructed: created from the contingent judgements about the adverse or undesirable outcomes of choices made by human beings. These 'hazards' are then invoked discursively to support estimations of risk, risky behaviour and of the people who take the risks.

The first step in grasping what at first sight may appear counterfactual, comes in recognizing that – as Wells (1996: 6) puts it – the 'materialisation of a hazard' is the result of identifying 'undesired or adverse events'. Many years ago, my lesson with advanced driving instructor Alan Oates illustrated that. For Alan, everything on the road was a *hazard*. What I thought was just a milk truck or a pedestrian crossing, turned out to be a hazard. That was the way he thought, and the result was safe – some would say, boring – driving. 'You're a top gear man, you always want to get into top gear even when approaching hazards', said Alan. 'Safety must be the paramount consideration, even if you have to sacrifice a little time' (Fox 1984).

To explore this further, let me consider the issue of health workers and infected sharps in some detail. Let us accept that discarded needles and other sharps that may have been infected by blood products exist as real objects. In and of themselves, these objects do not constitute a *hazard*. They become *hazardous* under certain circumstances, principally if conditions arise such that they may come into contact with and pierce the skin of a person in their vicinity. And we know this event is hazardous, not through some 'natural' quality of this event, but because we appraise it as undesired or adverse, based on bodies of knowledge about blood and the risks of infection associated with various blood-borne diseases such as hepatitis B and HIV. This cycle is illustrated in Figure 6.2.

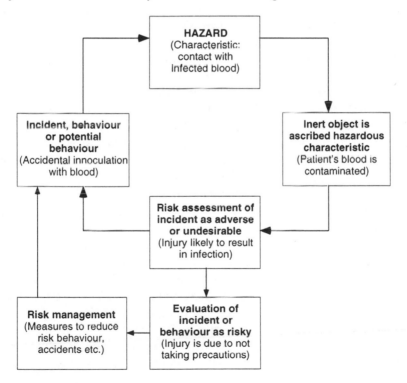

Figure 6.2 Risk assessment and the construction of hazards: contamination with infected blood

The transformation of an 'inert' object into one possessing *hazardous characteristics* (Wells 1996) thus occurs only as a result of our evaluations of *risk*, that is, the likelihood of an adverse result from an incident. Such evaluation may be based on anecdote or personal experience of danger or security. More formally, it may be based on a particular 'discourse' (an authoritative body of knowledge): that of risk assessment. Thus it is only in the analysis of *risks*, that the *hazard* comes into existence: if the risk is assessed as zero or close to zero, the inert object would remain just that (regardless of whether it 'really' does possess hazardous characteristics).

This model of hazard creation is at odds with received wisdom concerning the hazard/risk relationship. In Figure 6.1, hazards are prior to risks. What is argued now is that the selection of various 'inert' objects, procedures or humans as 'hazards' must itself depend upon some prior judgement, otherwise risk assessors would be faced with an insurmountable task of sifting through every element of an environment or context. Indeed, the impossibility of assessing every risk prospectively is reflected in the realities of risk analysis, which is sometimes faced with the consequences of a previously unidentified risk (Suter 1993: 313). Without some system of prioritization, analysis of risk would be absurdly long-winded, as analysts would forever be suggesting the most far-fetched, though potentially fatal, events to be avoided by safety precautions. Inevitably, risk assessment must begin with some prior knowledge about the world, what is 'probable' and what 'unlikely', what is 'serious', what is 'trivial' or seemingly 'absurd'. Such judgements may derive from 'scientific' sources, or may depend on 'common sense' or experiential resources; either way, the perception of a hazard's existence will depend on these judgements. How the judgement is made (that is, what is counted as evidence to support the assessment), is relative and culturally contingent.

This process of the construction of hazards can be seen in another study of health workers and contamination by blood, in which Grinyer explored 'expert' and 'lay' views on the prevention of accidental contact with blood products. While the hospital authorities issued guidelines to staff, needle-stick accidents had occurred, and staff were doubtful about how feasible it would be to avoid these incidents based on the guidelines. Grinyer found when she reported some accidents involving sharps and blood products, management denied her data's validity (1995: 40). She concluded that such unwillingness to recognize lay knowledge about hazards undermined risk reduction policies.

Not only are risk perceptions multi-dimensional, but, at any given time, people are managing a number of different agendas which may conflict with the official ones and can be contradictory. Official information is only one of a number of different routes through which a hazard is understood. Powerful social forces shape the way in which information is perceived and acted upon ... which may be underestimated by those responsible for risk assessment. (ibid.: 49)

Following Wynne, Grinyer argues that 'expertise' is often held by the lay actors, while expert knowledge is usually based only upon 'scientific evidence', and the latter is often privileged when it comes to what counts as a hazard (Wynne 1992: 285). In another study of risk assessment (of pesticide manufacture), Wynne suggested that

scientific risk analysis did not avoid, and could not have avoided, making social assumptions in order to create the necessary scientific knowledge. It was *conditional* knowledge in that its validity depended, *inter alia* upon the conditions in this embedded social model being fulfilled in actual practice. ... Each party, both scientists and workers, tacitly defined different actual risk systems. They built upon different models of the social practices controlling the contaminants and exposures. (Wynne 1992: 285–6 original emphases)

Wynne's argument is that technical or scientific discourses tend to make claims to objectivity while they tell the public how 'stupid and irrational they are' (1992: 286). This is not arrogance, but a failure by the 'experts' to recognize the contingency of their own position. Both sociologists and risk analysts have recognized that the credibility of evidence concerning whether an object is hazardous and the perceived 'relevance' of such evidence are weighed differently depending on perspective (Callon 1986, Suter 1993: 22, 40). This explains the failure of different groups to agree on risks: not because they interpret the data in different ways (the culturalist position set out earlier), but because they have different data: their differing knowledgeabilities prevent them from agreeing on what is to count as evidence of a hazard. It is not just outlooks on *risks* that are dependent on social milieu, but also world-views on *hazards* themselves. *Both risks and hazards are cultural products.*

What I am saying here is not that bad things do not happen as a result of certain incidents. However, it is necessary to emphasize this contingency of what is to be considered hazardous. Suter (1993) points out that human health cannot be taken as the 'gold standard' for environmental risk analysis, as this assumes that human health equates with biological protection more generally. Even if human health is taken as a standard, its applicability is not absolute: for the executioner, the lethal characteristics of electricity or narcotics are not *hazards*, they are the functional characteristics to be exploited. In such circumstances, a lethal outcome is not adverse or undesirable for all concerned: the incident is 'real', its hazardousness depends upon point of view.

Unlike the previous analyses, in which hazards are assumed to be the 'natural' underpinning of cultural attributions of risk, in this postmodern position the 'risky' quality of the environment is constructed from prospective assessment of the circumstances under which objects become hazardous (see Figure 6.2). Such predictions both establish 'hazards' and may create a subjectivity in people of being 'at risk' (and evaluations of which behavioural choices are 'safe' and which are 'risky'). In the rest of this chapter, I shall use this postmodern understanding of risk and hazard to explore issues of choice, first in relation to health at work and second to the use of the drug Ecstasy. Before that, I shall look in some detail at the issue of 'health' itself, which necessarily underpins any perspective on behaviour in relation to risks to health.

Risk and Arché-health

Were health an absolute, then the creation of a subjectivity which would tend to encourage 'healthy' living (i.e. behaviour minimizing health risks) could be accepted as non-problematic. However, as this book argues throughout, what 'health' is depends upon one's point of view. Notions of risk not only depend on an absolutism, but also bolster just such a view.

We saw earlier the moral dimension to attributions of 'risk', which are generally seen as the negative pole of an opposition to a desired state of 'safety'. Such moral positions are political, in that they ascribe rights and responsibilities to those subjected to them, and require actions in line with these rights or responsibilities. The human subject of risk analysis is drawn into a *subjectivity* as 'risky' and perhaps culpable. Similarly, any definition of health (be it medical or sociological) has a politics associated with it, inasmuch as it seeks to persuade us to a particular perspective on the person who is healthy or ill.

Modernism, it has been argued, is a project of *mastery* which begins with a process of definition and then – through reason and via the application of technology – controls and changes a phenomenon (typically, in this case, from 'ill' to 'healthy'). But recall the perspective on the nomadic subject which was developed in chapter 5, which suggests a way of rejecting territorialization into one way of being, and substituting a becoming-other. This might be considered as the basis for an ethics and politics (and I will have more to say on this in the final chapter of the book), based upon the celebration of difference and what White (1991) calls a *responsibility to otherness*. By this he means an engagement with others which encourages differentiation rather than prescribing a particular value against which the other should be evaluated.

In relation to issues of 'health' and 'illness', a responsibility to otherness suggests a radically different kind of response to others from that entailed by a biomedical or even biopsychosocial notion of health. Differentiation and transformation are involved, so rather than a static notion of human 'being', this kind of engagement is concerned with potential: with 'human becoming'. I coined the term *arché-health* (Fox 1993a) to denote this sense of health as concerned with 'becoming other' or transformation.

Arché-health is a process not a state, which – in its commitment to 'becoming-other' or transformation – resists attempts to impose a unifying identity (e.g. patient, man, foreigner, wife) on a thing or a person. It is most explicitly *not* an alternative model of health, or some prior state upon which concepts of health and illness are imposed. Rather it refers to the differences and the diversities which enable us to generate the ideas of 'health' and 'illness', terms which *can* reflect the dynamic, fluctuating character of the organism but which all too often are recruited as static conceptions which codify and evaluate that organism.

As a process of differentiation and transformation, *arché-health* (which is at the same time *arché-illness*) dissolves the opposition health/illness, offering in its place a flux and a multiplication of meaning. *Arché-health* can be seen in the active choice-making behaviour of people as they engage with their bodies, their bodies' functions and the efforts of doctors to normalize those functions. For carers, as I suggested in previous chapters, it is the process of reaching out to others, opening up possibilities and choices which a disease or disability closes down.

In sociological analysis, the notion of choice is unfashionable, perhaps even regarded as politically incorrect and reactionary. Both Marxist and Weberian traditions emphasized the constraints on action to be experienced by agents, while we have seen how a Foucauldian understanding of the construction of the self delineates a human subject seemingly incapable of resistance. In contrast, the kinds of perspectives developed in this book, using the work of such writers as Derrida, Deleuze and Guattari and Cixous, articulate with the notion of *arché-health* as a resistance to stasis or a becoming.

Risks – and particularly health risks – are intimately tied up with choices (Hertz and Thomas 1983: 3). If we acknowledge the constructed nature of 'health', then the subjectivity which arises from a definition of health is based in a partial truth grounded in some claim or other concerning what it is to be a human being, or have a body, or be part of a community, or whatever. This is where choice comes in, although not in an individualistic, rational-actor sense, implying a voluntaristic model of action. Rather, choice may be exerted negatively, in a refusal or resistance, as well as positively in affirmations. Choices may be temperamental or unconscious, or collective, as opposed to rational or individual. But such choosing is processual, and associated with *arché-health* in that it is a becoming rather than a state of being. I will illustrate this argument concerning risk and choice with two examples.

Health Risks and Choices at Work

Here is an extract from my study of surgical work (Fox 1992), and the hazards of blood-transmitted infection. A consultant surgeon Mr T and I talked during a procedure which, he had indicated, involved risks from the patient's blood.

> *Mr T:* Never a month goes by that we don't nick ourselves with a scalpel or other instrument, and I suppose we should be concerned about the risk, but we don't generally do anything.
> *Researcher:* I suppose the gloves offer some protection?
> *Mr T:* Yes, once a week I tear a glove, so they may help.
> *Researcher:* Do you take precautions when you have a patient who might be a risk?
> *Mr T:* Well, it's only if there is inoculation of blood that it's a problem.
> *Researcher:* What about blood spray into the eyes?
> *Mr T:* That can be a danger, I suppose. I often wear lenses (binocular magnifiers) so they have a double use. (Fox 1992: 29)

Mr T, as with other surgeons studied, seemed quite casual about hazards present in his work environment. He could take various actions to reduce these if he wished but all had costs associated with them (not do the procedures, invoke complicated precautions which would inhibit his freedom to operate as he wished). Ultimately he made choices to continue to do a job that he wanted to do, trying to take extra care where he perceived a higher risk. Work for Mr T was not simply something into which he was coerced, it was the result of a series of choices which he and his associates made on a daily basis.

Conversations with an operating department manager added support to this understanding. While nursing students and nursing auxiliaries needed counselling concerning health risks, this informant told me, 'higher-grade' staff were able to cope with risks because of their 'professionalism'. Thus the choices made by grades of nursing staff were based on their different perspectives on their work and responsibilities to others. Similarly, Mr T was *active* in his living out of a set of activities which are called 'work' and which impinged upon certain facets of the continuity of that life called 'health'. He made positive and negative choices concerning how he acted and how he saw himself in relation to his work setting and his associates and patients. His evaluations of hazards were based in these complex choices and perceptions, weighings of costs and benefits, and were part of his continual becoming-other: the *arché-health* of his unfolding life.

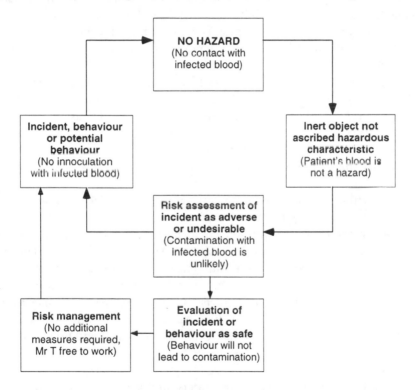

Figure 6.3 Mr T's reassessment of the risks and hazards of contamination with infected blood

For Mr T to be able to define his 'health' in this much broader sense of being free to choose how he lives and works, he redefined the hazards which his choices might lead him to encounter. His choice to work with patients others might see as 'high risk' resists the kind of cycle of hazard construction set out in Figure 6.2: he does not wish to accept the judgement that his behaviour is risky, as this would limit his actions. But if he assesses the risks involved as low (perhaps drawing on evaluations of his skill and the use of protection as evidence), the infectious body's hazardous characteristics are minimized, the hazard evaporates and it becomes more or less an inert object again (see Figure 6.3).

Risks, Choices and the Use of Ecstasy

The recreational drug MDMA, commonly known as Ecstasy, E or X, and used world-wide by millions of people as a mood enhancer, has been associated with a number of fatalities and a range of other less serious health consequences. Its relative newness as a street drug also means that long-term consequences of its use are unknown: it has been linked to chronic changes in neurotransmitter activity and certain other morbidities (Green and Goodwin 1996). While the death rate from acute affects cannot be easily calculated due to lack of figures about usage, most users will be aware of well-reported cases of deaths following use of Ecstasy. Supporters of the drug counter such stories, arguing that risks are small, and usually associated with the context of ingestion rather than the drug itself. Thus the independent researcher Saunders suggests:

> To say that a person died from Ecstasy is never the full story any more than saying that someone died of drink: like alcohol, Ecstasy can be used without any harmful effect. In both cases, death is due to the indirect effects which can be avoided if you are aware of the dangers and look after yourself. The difference is that the dangers of being drunk are well known and recognised, while the dangers resulting from Ecstasy use are far less known. Far from saving young people from harm, much of the so-called drugs education has confused users by trying to scare them, rather than explain the dangers and how to avoid them. (Saunders 1995)

I am not concerned to debate the 'safety' of Ecstasy, nor with how statistics are used to argue for or against its use. Rather, I am interested to see how users evaluate this evidence, and what affects the choices of hundreds of thousands of people to use Ecstasy on a regular basis. The reason for choosing this example derives from the unequivocal evidence that pure MDMA (that is, Ecstasy which has not been cut with other drugs or toxic substances) produces a highly pleasurable experience. For instance, one respondent on a web site devoted to the study of Ecstasy commented

The Ecstasy was *unbelievable* and the music was even better. The people there were lovely, the vibe was alive and growing! I spent the night in heaven, meeting people, hugging and dancing my brains out. ... I was moved into such a deep state of trance, the music, the lights, the vibe from the beautiful girl dancing across from me ... it was perfect!

Ecstasy offers the possibility of a release from the alienation of everyday life.

We were liberated from the chains that bound us for that night. It was an experience of absolute freedom. We danced, talked, laughed and revelled with the world. When we arrived home at night, we gathered in the family room and spoke to the camcorder. The next day when we watched the video we could not believe how different we seemed – so relaxed, happy and natural. Why couldn't life always be like this?

The following responses indicate the kinds of judgements used by those taking the drug for the first time

I am a 30-year-old first time trier, having resisted the influence to do so for all my 20s on the basis that I was too old and it would be unnecessary/dangerous to do so. What bollocks. I stayed up all night with no fatigue and great enjoyment both emotionally, socially, physically and a little spiritually.

I researched this drug before I did it to find out as much as I could about its possible side effects, dangers, other people's experiences, good or bad, everything that I thought might help me in my decision, and made a decision to do it. I believe that knowing what I was doing and going into it with a positive outlook and in an environment that I was comfortable in helped this to be the transforming experience that it was for me.

The night that we took the E, I was feeling very stressed out and in a bad mood. I had told my older brother and his wife what I was planning to do, and they had some very harsh criticisms to offer as they felt that it was dangerous. I personally did not know much about E, but I trusted my boyfriend S who had done a lot of research on the topic and was careful about what he put into our bodies.

These comments could be read as lay risk assessments and in a sense that is what they are. Gillian Taberner's research (personal communication) supports the premise that what is happening here is an active choice-making concerning the possibilities facing these users: each is weighing the desirable outcomes of taking the drug against negative consequences. Her informant Andrew said:

> People are becoming more open-minded about it because a lot of people are taking it. Virtually everybody knows someone who takes Ecstasy or has taken it and they're still alive, still having a good time.

Such choices are processual, continually rethought. Another respondent, Zoe, wondered

> Do you think when you get older you get, like I think I'll get more concerned about my body as well. It feels like when you're young it's OK because you've got control over most things but when you're older you think ...

When the risks outweigh the attractions, Ecstasy becomes a *hazard*, while for those respondents who decide to take the drug, its possible hazardousness is sidelined, and the drug is seen as an opportunity to experience a desired state.

In the previous section I discussed the surgeon's *arché-health*: the becoming-other which resulted from his active choice-making. Similarly, we can see the choices made by these users of Ecstasy as a manifestation of their *arché-health*. Ecstasy is an integral part of the lives of many young people (Power *et al*. 1996: 78) and to take it is to experience a highly desired set of consequences. The choices of people to use E reflect a desire to incorporate the experiences available through using the drug, or to affirm particular facets of users' self-identity (Beck and Rosenbaum 1994). To perceive Ecstasy as a hazard is not part of the world-view of those positively inclined toward its psychological effects: instead it is a means to a highly rated objective. The bias of pro-Ecstasy commentators in assessing the evidence of risk reflects this differing world-view: one in which the spiritual and psychological highs of Ecstasy use far outstrip the risks identified by medical researchers (Rushkoff 1994, Jordan 1995). Buchanan's research on teenagers' perceptions of drugs supports this. Notions of harm or illegality are relatively insignificant for many users: 'whether or not drug use is harmful, and/or whether it is against the law, the more important and overriding concern for those at high risk appears to be the issue of individual choice' (Buchanan 1991: 330–1).

Those who would control the use of Ecstasy must therefore recognize the impact that it has upon the subjectivity of users, and how far the psychological, emotional and spiritual attractiveness of a drug counters perceived risks (Amos *et al.* 1997). This point is important, because while the decision by a surgeon to operate despite objective assessments of risk from infection may be seen as altruistic and laudable, the decisions of people to use substances which have risks associated with them are more likely to be judged as foolhardy and culpable. In both cases, this analysis suggests a perspective which emphasizes choice, but in the case of Ecstasy use, this kind of analysis is less likely to be favoured. My point, however, is the same for both situations: that people's behaviour must be seen not as based upon differential judgements of risk, but within the context of world-views which may deviate very greatly from that of the 'expert' risk assessor.

Risks and Opportunities

I have used two disparate examples in this chapter to unpack the constructed nature of hazards. They were chosen to illustrate the active process of becoming which is part of human lives in settings which may seem very different: comparing the relatively constrained arena of work with the relatively unconstrained leisure context of illegal drug use.

The intention has been to suggest a way of thinking about the hazard/risk dichotomy which is not supplied in either the 'realist' or 'culturalist' perspectives. While building on the insights of the culturalist position (that risks are culturally constructed), it moves beyond what might thus be seen as a culture/nature opposition. In the 'postmodern' position, risks are not absolutes, but neither are the 'hazards' which are supposedly the circumstances which constitute risks. It turns out that the supposedly natural phenomena of hazards are constructed through the lens of culture. This position bears some resemblance to Woolgar's (1988) argument that even such 'natural entities' as subatomic particles and the continent of America are 'invented' rather than 'discovered' inasmuch as the concepts are produced in a social process and satisfy certain cultural requirements in order to be accepted as real. The position developed from post-structuralism, with its emphasis on *textual* construction of reality, is more sceptical about a direct relationship between cultural contexts and the natural entities which are constructed, acknowledging the intertextual character of such reality construction, which is both complex and always an unfinished project (Curt 1994: 36). What is hazardous is often likely to be highly contested, and the kinds of situations concerning hazard assessment explored by Wynne (1992) bear this out.

If the very character of the environment in which we live (and this includes our bodies) is constructed in texts, and these texts are contested between different 'authorities', risk analysis is a deeply political activity. The identification of hazards (and the consequent definition of what is a risk), can easily lead to the valorization of certain kinds of living over others. In a 'risk society', notions of health and work will be – in part – dependent upon what is seen as a risk or a hazard. Social perceptions of health and work will in turn contribute to the on-going construction of 'risk' itself. We implicitly evaluate certain actions or situations in terms of the consequences for others or ourselves and label these actions or situations as more or less threatening to our physical, psychological or moral integrity.

'Risk', like 'health', is a concept which contributes to how we think about modern life. These concepts are tied up with the values of a culture and the moral rights and responsibilities of members of that culture, and as such are implicated in how people understand themselves as reflexive, ethical subjects. Because these conceptions are contingent, the subjectivities which are created around risk, health and work are also relative: if this means that we are constrained by cultural constructions of subjectivity, it also means we can resist. The analysis which has been offered in this chapter offers a perspective on 'risk-taking' as the active process of choosing as life unfolds: a *becoming-other* and a resistance to discourse. In a somewhat different context, and harking back to my work on older adults' experiences of care, the group *Counsel and Care* has argued that because a person is living in a protective environment, that does not diminish the human right to take risks (Counsel and Care 1993: section 2, page 1). Such a notion of a human right is essentialist, but it may be argued similarly that the autonomy of the human individual – within or without the workplace – cannot be simply denied because she or he is apparently behaving in a way judged to be risky. The implications of such a position are that it is neither sufficient to point to phenomena and claim they are hazardous (because such claims are always dependent upon the partial evidence deemed relevant by the claimant), nor to assume that by making such claims one is necessarily acting in the interests of those who one may be trying to assist.

I have been concerned in this chapter to establish the basis upon which people may resist authoritative statements about how humans should behave. This postmodern perspective on risks and hazards is not intended to challenge the critiques of industrial production as often injurious to the bodies, minds and spirits of individuals. However, it does suggest that 'health' should be understood as constituted in the unfolding lives of individuals with their own choice-making agendas for living and dying. The *becoming-other* of body, mind or spirit is processual: differently formulated and in the right circumstances, a *risk* to 'health' can be an *opportunity* for transformation and renewal.

Whatever is beyond health is not *arché-health*, because *arché-health* is not a 'thing' but rather the system of difference which makes possible the continually unfolding possibilities of a nomadic subjectivity. Deleuze and Guattari speak of smooth space (of which, more in chapter 8) as the realm of the nomad (1988: 353). In opposition to the striated space of the territorialized subject (which is where we all live almost all of the time), smooth space is dimensionless, a place in which a nomad can wander (ibid.: 479–81). Yet wandering is perhaps the wrong word as it suggests aimlessness. There is a passage in *A Thousand Plateaus* which is particularly evocative of what it is to be a nomad in smooth space:

> We can say of the nomads ... *they do not move*. They are nomads by dint of not moving, not migrating, of holding a smooth space that they refuse to leave, that they leave only in order to conquer and die. Voyage in place ... Voyaging smoothly is a becoming, and a difficult, uncertain becoming at that. (ibid.: 482).

Voyaging in smooth space is not only difficult and uncertain, it is also – by definition – impossible to generalize. I cannot tell you how to become a nomad, any more than I can be told by you. But I have suggested some tools. First, it is clear that it entails deconstructive activity, indeed deconstruction is nomadology. Second, it is not something which has to be a solitary activity: the other may be crucial in supplying a crucial gift which makes all the difference in deterritorialization, even if it is a gift the other does not realize she or he is giving (Derrida 1993). Third, it is processual: we live out our lives in the pursuit of smooth space, and perhaps it can never be reached so long as we are trapped in our language and our concepts. Yet these features of being human, of being able to use language to abstract, deconstruct and reconstruct, are also the means for deterritorialization. Finally, it is a practical activity: one in which theory is of use only to resist, not to control. It is to this issue that I now turn.

7
Research and/as Nomadology

The Truth is Not Out There

As I indicated at the outset of this project, the prime motivation for this book is to inform practice: the practical activities of individuals seeking a nomadic movement *beyond health*, and of practitioners involved in the areas of health and social care. This emphasis is both a feature of the subject area, and is grounded in a political commitment to overturn a privileging of the 'academic', in the sense of that word that implies the codifying and regulation of action and practice. Indeed, readers may have discerned a thread running through this book which is critical of the academic underpinning of practice. For example, in chapter 3 it was argued that care-as-profession is based in a disciplinary apparatus which controls and imposes definitions upon its subjects. Then, in the previous chapter, notions of risk and risky behaviour developed by health and social science disciplines were deconstructed, to emphasize the choice-making behaviour of individuals, and the disciplinary nature of 'risk' itself.

Does this critique mean that all efforts to theorize and understand the social world are to be rejected as adjuncts of this process of disciplinary limitation, based on the 'academic encirclement' of human behaviour? In other words, should we abandon all efforts to use science and rationality to make sense of the world about us? Should this even be taken as an antagonism to theory? In terms of the critique of modernism which has been put forward here and elsewhere (for example, Fox 1993a, Game 1991), it could be argued that this is precisely what should happen. In a kind of postmodern flurry of relativism, we would be thrust back into a medievalism, in which there was no longer any recourse to the scientific method, including the use of observation and concomitant theory-building.

I believe that there is an alternative to this very radical proposition, and in this chapter, I wish to develop a more thought-out postmodern (as opposed to some kind of return to the pre-modern) perspective on knowledge, truth and research. I will start by setting out the bare bones of the modernist perspective on research and then develop a number of themes which can offer an alternative model for research which is within the spirit of the arguments developed in the rest of this book concerning nomadology. As will be seen, this nomadological or nomadic approach to research dissolves the practice/research dichotomy along with a number of other dualisms relevant to health and embodiment.

It is hardly news that the postmodern position rejects the modernist view that knowledge can be gleaned about the world around us in such a way that we can – in theory at least – get to 'truth'. Modernism is synonymous with the scientific methodologies of observation and inductive reasoning from the particular observation to a general proposition about the world. Indeed, it is a fundamental of modernity that the world can be made comprehensible through science and rationality: this modernist *hubris* is both part of the spirit of the scientific age and, as we shall see in a moment, highly normative. These commitments underpin and make possible the enterprise of 'research' in a modernist sense, and it is worth considering how this enterprise has been constituted. The two notions of internal and external validity provide a straightforward way into this critique.

First, modernism applies a scientific *logocentrism*. Logocentrism, for Derrida (1978), amounts to the claim that by one route or another, it is possible to achieve truth or the *logos* – unmediated knowledge of the world. Logocentrisms underpin many systems of thought, from religion and cultural assumption through logic and deductive reasoning to – most recently – science. If only, the argument goes, our methodology is adequate and appropriate, then we will be able to achieve an understanding based upon the observations that we make and the theory we develop to explain those observations. Scientific logocentrism – while on the one hand privileging research data gathered through specified methods – downgrades the 'mere experience' which is developed in practical settings (Wood *et al.* 1998: 1730).

Each scientific discipline has adapted its logocentrism to meet the beliefs about how knowledge may be gleaned, and neophytes within a science must learn the rules of their particular game. Once these rules are established, the findings about the word gained from research are reified as truth, and as Kuhn (1962) points out, a scientific community often considers anomalous research findings not as true deviations from accepted beliefs about the world but as failures of method. Methods texts can be seen as science's equivalent of a religion's holy book: setting out the right way to do things, and the 'threats to validity' which come from not following the prescriptions and precedents. These rules about method are summed up in the traditional notion of 'internal validity', which is concerned with determining that a study measures what it set out to measure. (It is worth noting that behind debates about methodology there are more fundamental issues of epistemology – philosophical questions about how it is possible to know. For the social sciences, methodological arguments are often played out at this level. Thus for example, in sociology, positivism and naturalistic perspectives have argued the toss, while more recently, realism and postmodern approaches have taken issue over questions of representation in social enquiry. The continuing 'crisis' of modernism rests in its increasing acknowledgement that the holy grail of unmediated knowledge is slipping away: knowledge will always be mediated by observation. From quantum physics to social theory, it is recognized that the observer irrevocably affects what is observed.)

The second element of this perspective is related to the 'external validity' of research, concerning the generalizability of research findings to practical settings. Particularly in biomedical research and randomized controlled trials, it often seems as if the research process ends when the analysis has been completed and the paper submitted for publication. This ignores the whole issue of the translation of research into practical settings (Callon 1986, Wood *et al.* 1998).

Recently – especially in health and medicine – there has been an emphasis upon 'evidence-based practice', meaning practice which has been underpinned by scientific explorations to establish patterns and truths about the world. Thus for example, health professionals should manage their patients according to guidelines based on research evidence rather than drawing upon their own experiences or depending on what they learnt from their teachers. This philosophy emphasizes the need for rational and research-based practical activities. The regular failure of research findings to be translated into practice is then blamed on the practitioners, who are assumed to be either recalcitrant or incapable of adapting the research which informs their practical setting. I will devote space at the end of this chapter to an appraisal of this phenomenon from a postmodern perspective on knowledge.

Traditionally, the modernist perspective has privileged modes of research that can provide quantifiable data, perhaps reflecting the roots of modernity in accounting practice (Weber 1971, Fox 1991). Qualitative data and case studies are sometimes seen as 'first steps' in gaining understanding, to be followed up by more 'rigorous' and 'systematic' methods, often entailing hypothesis testing by means of inferential statistical analysis. Even disciplines such as sociology which have embraced qualitative methods limit the claims to be made about research findings generated from such approaches (see for example, Lincoln and Guba's (1985) discussion of generalizability or external validity of qualitative data). Such a view rejects the value of contingent knowledge such as may exist in one setting but not in another. In Weberian terms, this is to confuse *formal* rationality concerned with the calculability of means and procedures, with *substantive* rationality – the situated and contingent evaluation of ends or results (Brubaker 1984: 36, Fox 1991: 714).

The postmodern critique of these elements is based on the view that there is not one single 'truth' about the world. That is not to say that we cannot possess knowledge of the world, but rather that there are a number of 'truths' which are historically- and setting-contingent. It acknowledges complexity and diversity, rather than seeking patterns and overarching 'grand narratives'. Modernism, it may be said, has a world-view which *denies difference*, seeking to define and compartmentalize. In contrast, postmodernism might be said to be committed to and *constitutive of difference* (Haber 1994: 13). It refuses to create hierarchies or construct reductive frameworks for meaning. This principle of difference will be central to the discussion when I turn to consider postmodern research later in this chapter.

In terms of internal validity, postmodernism rejects the view that there is one best way to achieve knowledge of the world, because it rejects the notion of unmediated knowledge. All knowledge must depend not only upon the setting, but also upon who is doing the observation, and under what circumstances. Methodology filters out the randomness of the world, and imposes an invisible discipline on knowledge and truth. In terms of external validity, the same arguments apply: there is little possibility of becoming context-independent. Consequently, it is unlikely that research findings can be generalized beyond the setting in which they were gathered.

At the beginning of this chapter I said I wanted to reject a postmodern approach to research which denied the possibility of any knowledge of the world. From what has just been suggested concerning internal and external validity, it could also be argued that the watchwords of postmodern research would be 'anything goes', and indeed, an eclecticism may be attractive as one element of encouraging difference. Furthermore, we must accept that there are many differing postmodernisms, with different perspectives and concomitant consequences for thinking about knowledge (Rosenau 1992). However, in the spirit of what has gone before in this book, and specifically with an interest in Deleuze and Guattari's work, in the following section I will develop the postmodern critique in a particular direction. I shall start by considering some of the features of Deleuze and Guattari's nomadology, to suggest one kind of postmodern research. Addressing key stages in the modernist research process, I will suggest an alternative *nomadic research* which acknowledges the impossibility of gaining unmediated knowledge or truth, yet offers possibilities for practice informed by exploration and explanatory modelling of the setting.

The Detective and the Nomad Revisited

It is appropriate at this point to recall the distinction made in the introductory chapter of this book between the modernist icon of the detective and the postmodern nomad. This comparison was used to suggest the different ways in which modernism and postmodernism engage with and understand the world. The detective – as summed up in the figure of Sherlock Holmes – is a seeker after truth, using observation and deduction to make sense of and explain the world around him or herself. This modernist icon is grounded in a *will to mastery* (White 1991) and a humanist expectation that all will be revealed through the power of human reason (Carroll 1993). The nomad, on the other hand, has a different engagement with the world. As has been suggested in previous chapters, the nomad does not seek control or mastery of the environment, but rather, passes through it stopping here and there and wherever. She or he takes what is useful, but always with the recognition that after an hour or a month or ten years it will be time to move on. Unlike the modernist detective, who enhances the *striation* (Deleuze and Guattari 1988: 353) of the environment by the naming of this, that and the other in her constant search for explanation and truth, the nomad inhabits a *smooth space*. Paradoxically, she celebrates difference, not by differentiating, but by accepting every aspect of the environment as being of equal value. No place, setting or time is privileged over another – all are equivalent and of equal significance. Nor is movement privileged over stasis: it is possible to be nomadic and never move!

The icon of the detective is an avatar for the modernist researcher with her commitment to truth through reason and the scientific enterprise. Given the very different positions which the detective and the nomad hold in relation to the world, it is unsurprising – if this metaphor holds – that research in postmodern mood will also differ widely from the traditional modern form, both in terms of methods and procedures and of underpinning epistemological and ontological standpoints. From the arguments developed earlier in this book, it is easy to suggest some of the features by which research as nomadology will be characterized.

First, pursuit of knowledge must be recognized to be a *local and contingent* process. While understanding of the environment may be achieved through observation and inductive reasoning, it cannot be assumed that these observations or this reasoning can be translated to other settings, or even from the research setting to 'real life'. Indeed, a commitment to the celebration of difference requires that no such assumptions be made.

Second, as with all actions, research activity should be *constitutive of difference*, rather than constitutive of identity. Unlike the modernist will to mastery, which pigeonholes phenomena into categories based on their qualities or hierarchical positioning in relation to each other, the nomadic celebration of difference smooths out these striations. It acknowledges different qualities, yet accepts them as of equal value rather than hierarchically or oppositionally privileged in relation to each other. Thus, for example, as we saw in the previous chapter, 'risky behaviour' is not privileged over 'safe behaviour', rather these different actions are seen as equally legitimate choices of human agents. Similarly, nomadic research would avoid legitimating or repressing particular aspects of the world it observes.

Third, *theory building* – while necessarily part of any activity of 'understanding' – should be seen not as an end in itself but as an *adjunct to practical activity* within the setting in question. In particular, there would be an avoidance of meta-narratives (Lyotard 1984) or grand theory, which seeks to globalize and deny difference. The value of theory will be in its applicability in immediate practical activities in settings in which it has been developed. Understanding makes sense only if data are placed in context (Mauthner *et al.* 1998).

It is possible to build a model of postmodern research with the benefit of these three propositions, and later in the chapter I shall do just that. But I want to proceed in a less linear manner, to wander and meander in nomadic mood. First, I shall explore some relevant strands: issues of reflexivity and the multiplication of meaning which derive from the *intertextual* character of our understandings, the model of knowledge acquisition known as *action research*, and – along the way – more general issues of the *ethics and politics* of an engaged research.

Reflexivity, Intertextuality and Knowledge

Reflexivity and intertextuality are tied up with the same phenomenon: the continual meaning ascription which human beings engage in as they apprehend and construct the world and their own senses of self (Game 1991). While both are inevitable features of a linguistically mediated culture, reflexivity and intertextuality are only now being recognized as central to the process of representation which is involved in gaining knowledge about the world. Reflection has been advocated not only in the more 'private' realms of life to help people understand more about themselves, but as an adjunct to professional and organizational development (Winter 1989). However, for the purposes of evaluating the contribution to the research process, I shall explore the issue of reflexivity through its partner: intertextuality.

Intertextuality is the process whereby one text (taken in the widest sense of any culturally-produced object or social practice capable of being understood) plays upon other texts. Intertextually, texts refer endlessly to further elements within the realm of cultural production (Barthes 1977). Thus the film *Apocalypse Now* relates intertextually to other texts including Conrad's *Heart of Darkness* and many other films and books about wars in south-east Asia. Road signs or a set of traffic signals connects a driver to a text such as the British *Highway Code* or other manuals on road safety. In this book the references are intertextual links to other bodies of work, which in turn lead to other texts and so on, *ad infinitum*.

Every text has an 'intertext' of related texts for a reader (even if this is limited to a dictionary), and the 'chaining of signification' from one text to another can easily be used to consciously enhance and emphasize the open-endedness of textuality and 'knowledge'. Focusing on intertextuality can contribute a rereading of the relationships between the world, the observer, the writer and the reader, between researchers and researched, students and teachers, theorists and practitioners. Through this process of reflection, intertextuality is a means to challenge and resist the limits of a system of thought: to open up the possibilities of becoming other (Bogue 1989, Curt 1994, White 1991).

Within the frame of postmodern theory, an interest in writing and intertextuality rejects distinctions between real and representation (Stanley and Morgan 1993: 3). All texts, in this view, are fabrications, and as such are subject to deconstructive rewriting and rereading. Research texts, like any others, are to be read and reread, not as representations (accurate or flawed) of the world, but as contested claims to speak 'the truth' about the world, constituted in the play of disciplines of the social. Research writing, in this model, becomes narrative work (Maines 1993: 17).

Sciences have gained legitimacy (although not incontestably) for their particular claims to knowledge of reality in the modern period. But this *logocentrism* on the part of science works only by a denial (or bracketing) of other competing claims: as such, it is also a denial of intertextuality. Recognition of the intertext is implicitly a critique of logocentrism. It challenges science's privilege to speak authoritatively about the world (to paraphrase Game (1991: 18), science's fiction is that science is not fiction). But, I would suggest that at the same time, this analysis *opens up* the possibilities for a research practice which is no longer obsessed by efforts to attain some kind of transparent mediation of knowledge of the world by the human observer (Flax 1990, Hutcheon 1989). If no privilege is attached to particular discourses, 'researchers' may explore far more widely texts which contribute to the fabrication of the world. In short, it proffers a new richness of 'data' from the play of text on text in novel and unending combinations.

I want to suggest here that *intertextuality* is a feature of the deterritorialization of subjectivity and nomadism which underpins the theory of resistance developed earlier in this book. Deleuze and Guattari make this explicit in *A Thousand Plateaus* (1988), recognizing the significance of the intertext: it is a book designed as a 'rhizome' to be read hypertextually – in any order, refusing to follow a single chain of signification (1988: 7–9, see also Landow 1992 for a discussion of hypertext and postmodernism). Their objective – perhaps – is to orchestrate enough intensities upon the reader's BwO that new connections become possible, a new plateau is achieved, so the reader can say 'so that's what it's about'. Deleuze and Guattari's book is also explicitly an incitement to write.

> Conjugate deterritorialized flows. Follow the plants: you start by delimiting a first line consisting of circles of convergence around successive singularities; then you see whether inside that line new circles of convergence establish themselves, with new points located outside the limits and in other directions. Write, form a rhizome, increase your territory by de-territorialization, extend the line of flight to the point where it becomes an abstract machine covering the entire plane of consistency. (1988: 11)

The argument that writing is one way to become other (echoed in a range of writings reviewed in Fox 1993a), suggests the possibilities that research can be turned from an academic activity into part of the on-going practice of choosing and becoming. I would like to illustrate the significance of such intertextuality for my own 'becoming' through a reflection on my research activities. During the late 1980s, I undertook an ethnography of surgery at a number of UK hospitals, which was later published (Fox 1992) as a monograph, and continued to be recycled in various forms as part of my efforts to explore postmodern social theory. A richness can be brought to this kind of writing of the social by exploring the play of a range of texts, in addition to the 'straight' ethnographic report which I originally produced in an effort to describe events in the operating theatre or on the surgical wards.

The first text I draw on in this exercise in intertextuality is the fabricated field notes which formed the basis of the ethnographic report. For example, take the extract reported in chapter 2 (p. 66) which formed part of a discussion of the organization of the surgical day. Extracts such as this formed the 'official' text in which I attempted to represent surgery. Methodologically, its claim to authority rested upon the representation of observations conducted during field-work. It is hardly necessary to make the point that the relationship between the observed and this account of it is the outcome of interpretative and representational work which renders it no more than a plausible fiction (Atkinson 1990, Tyler 1986). But, while I was writing up these notes, I was also reading a variety of texts which were relevant to the phenomena I was studying. Some, like Katz (1984) and Atkinson (1981), were social science ethnographies. But I was also reading fictional accounts of surgery, and the televising of Colin Douglas's book *The Houseman's Tale* – a medical romp in the spirit of *Doctor in the House* – coincided with the field-work. Here is an extract from another of Douglas's books: *Bleeders Come First* (1979).

> The nurse held Miss Warrender's arm back as Campbell gripped the wrist with both hands, palms downwards and pulled. There was an uneasy, crunchy feel as the ends of the fracture came apart, then he bent the wrist backwards and outwards a little and let the lower fragment of the broken bone settle gently back into place, or rather into what he hoped was its right place.
>
> There was soft tissue swelling round the site of the fracture, which made the result of his efforts harder to assess, but in general it was a better-looking wrist than it had been. The hollow and step had gone, and if there was any resemblance to an old-fashioned dinner fork, it was now only a very slight one.
>
> 'That might be it,' said Campbell. 'Like to feel it, nurse, before we put the slab on?'
>
> 'Yes please.' The nurse ran her fingers over the straightened forearm. 'I see.'
>
> The gasman, holding the mask on the patient's face with one hand, and keeping a finger on the carotid pulse in the neck at the same time, was beginning to look impatient. (1979: 89)

This fictional patient subsequently had a cardiac arrest on the operating table and died, despite having come to casualty for a very minor procedure. Such tales (and more recent visualizations such as the TV fictions *ER* and *Cardiac Arrest*), paradoxically, bring back to me more fully than my field notes some of the 'real-ness' of surgery, the blood, the smells of the operating theatre, and the tragedy of individual cases which go badly. Fictional writings bring together elements which do not necessarily coincide conveniently in ethnographic observations of 'reality'. Many of these elements – which fabricate that part of the social called surgery – are consequently lost in my official account. For instance, Douglas's text reminds me not to overlook the uncertainty involved in surgery and the unpredictability of patients' responses to surgical interventions. Such reminders serve as a counterpoint to the standard analyses of power imbalances and control in sociological readings of the medical, and offer further readings for the kinds of chaotic organization which I described (Fox 1992).

In traditional research, other elements are often submerged or denied. Look at a third text related to the study: part of my own field-work diary, which documented my impressions and thoughts during field-work, and in which I reflected on my own experience of sometimes distressing events, or merely the embarrassments of being a supernumerary. Here is an extract (which never got translated into ethnography) concerning an episode in neurosurgery.

> (Date label) After the fiasco yesterday I was relieved that everyone seemed to know who I was. The neuro-theatre complex had a very different feel to it – different layout from the others, and seems more cut off from the rest of the hospital. This needs working on. ... The case which followed really affected me. It was a boy of about 10 with a tumour on his brain, and some injury to his neck. He was in pain and was crying because he had been hurt while being brought from the Children's Hospital in an ambulance. It was really awful, and I walked out of the room until he was unconscious. This is the first operation on a child I have seen, and it made me realize what people go through in surgery. I cannot bring myself to write this up in the log, and don't know if I want to include it in the thesis.

And indeed, this case *was* never written.

I suggest that reading these various texts together supplies a new richness to the exploration of this aspect of the world. Many other texts could be introduced, and the process of intertextual reading is consequently never-ending. But for the sake of this short discussion, what can be made of the play of these three texts? Certainly something further in terms of 'evoking' (Tyler 1986) surgery is made available for reading and writing. But also, I can see here my desire to produce an objective account, my inability to cope with some of the emotional aspects of surgical care, maybe suppressing or excluding exploration of how surgical staff cope, a need to explore how staff engage with their patients. These readings are all available for fabrication, and they in turn constitute new texts – for instance: this one. The potency, for the writer or the reader, inheres in the possibility always to read another text, or to reread it in a new way. I talked about this issue in a paper at the British Sociological Association conference, and a further text exists in the form of a tape-recording I made of my presentation there. And I can read my efforts back then – to reintroduce a 'lost' emotional aspect of my research – as part of a more general recognition of the suppression of the emotional in my life, which I was facing up to at the time the conference paper was written. There can always be a further text.

What are the implications for research practice in opening up the range of texts which are considered 'legitimate' research data? First, intertextual approaches break the distinction between researcher and researched, inasmuch as the researcher becomes part of the world which is being explored and translated into text. The significance of the researcher's intertextual links in documenting the world must be recognized, and distinctions between the personal and professional responses of researchers in field settings are elided.

Second, researchers become part of an intertextuality such that they can no longer stand apart from their research setting: their relationship with 'subjects' must be acknowledged as part of a wider social and political engagement than simply of researcher/researched. Consequently, the researcher must adopt an ethical and political position which structures the engagement which she or he has with the subjects of research. A commitment to intertextuality is also a commitment to difference and to becoming other. The politics of intertextuality and the postmodern are radical and concerned with resistance and change.

Third, the significance of writing research reports changes from efforts to represent or to persuade, to a reflection upon the relationship between that text and other texts, to the possibilities of deterritorialization and nomadism. Researchers may choose a fictional genre in preference to factual accounts (for example Curt 1994, Mulkay 1985), where this seems to offer the greatest potential to challenge the established systems of thought and knowledge. At other times, texts in the form of a direct engagement (teaching, therapy, protest, worship) may be considered more appropriate than traditional forms of reporting research findings. Whatever form is chosen, intertextually the research becomes part of the setting it is exploring, and the ethics of research become inextricably tied up with the wider issues of political engagement, struggle and resistance to power and injustice.

Action Research: Towards an Ethically and Politically Engaged Research

The second thread which impinges upon the development of nomadic research is the methodology known as 'action research'. Action research has a fairly long history within the social sciences, and in particular educational research, yet it has been marginalized and is often ignored in methodology texts. Action research is usually traced back to the work of Kurt Lewin in organizational psychology, but has subsequently developed in a number of differing directions, each grounded in different philosophical and political commitments. An early manifestation of action research was the Fox projects, conducted in the US in the 1940s and 1950s. The principles of this research were to develop and test theory on an on-going basis in interaction with interventions or actions; ensure consistency between project means and desired ends; and base ends and means upon guidelines established by the host community (Stull and Schensul 1987).

This model of action or advocacy research may be discerned in a study by Schensul *et al.* (1987) which extended the use of a traditional model of maternal care into a new setting, in order to enhance child health. Such a model sustains the distinction between researcher and researched, while acknowledging the importance of accounting for the perspectives of the researched subjects. Another health-care example of this kind of approach may be found in Hart and Bond (1995). Similarly, Nixon (1981) describes a model of 'practitioner research' which is appropriate for teachers in classroom settings.

These three examples of action research fall into the first of three categories set out by Carr and Kemmis (1986). Action research, they argued could be classed as

(a) technical (in which an outside expert undertakes the research);
(b) practical (in which the researched are encouraged to participate in the research process); and
(c) emancipatory (in which the researcher takes on the role of a 'process moderator' assisting participants to undertake the research themselves).

The third of these models is of the most interest for exploring the nomadic approach to research, and has been adopted by a number of educational researchers. For example, Zuber-Skerritt suggests that within this paradigm, action research is practical, participative and collaborative, emancipatory, interpretive and critical. Reflective practitioners undertake critical evaluation, are accountable and make results public. In this way, 'action and practical experience may be the foundations of ... research, and research may inform practice and lead to action' (Zuber-Skerritt 1991: 11).

Emancipatory action research has been associated with critical theory, and is predicated on political commitments to participation and improvement in quality of life among participants. Carr and Kemmis emphasize the importance of reflexivity, such that theory and practice, thought and action are related dialectically. From a Habermasian position, they conceive of a 'self-critical' community of action researchers who are committed to the improvement of practice (1986: 184). Considering the benefits of collaborative research, Schensul (1987) suggests that it can

(a) bring together people with diverse skills and knowledge;
(b) de-mystify the research process, allowing practitioners to shape the data collection process;
(c) build a research capacity into a community which can operate independently;
(d) increase the likelihood of the use of research findings by practitioners; and
(e) improve the quality of research by enabling access to key bodies of knowledge in a community.

Stonach and MacLure push this elision of the researcher and researched further. In their postmodern perspective on educational research, they suggest that the 'researcher' is a construction, nothing more than 'an effect of a representational economy, a false unity or a representational fix' (1997: 100). They are attracted to the concept of a 'transgressive validity' for research, as outlined earlier by Laller (1993). In this perspective, the validity of research is a function of its capacity to transgress, challenge or subvert existing conceptions. However, Stonach and MacLure (1997) note that within the spirit of transgressive validity, this concept would necessarily be subject to transgression itself. As has already been suggested, 'validity' depends on evaluations of research against some standard, and in the kind of localized and contingent postmodern perspective developed here, no such standards may be sustained.

However, a model of 'transgressive research' is not problematic in quite the same way, inasmuch as what is implied by this term is research which – as has been proposed earlier as one principle of nomadic research – is constitutive of difference. In addition to the principles underpinning emancipatory action research – namely, of reflexivity and collaboration, transgressive research has a commitment to challenge norms and assumptions, resisting power and constraint and opening up new possibilities. While many of the processes which would be involved in undertaking research of this kind would be similar to those of the 'emancipatory' action research (Carr and Kemmis 1986), transgressive research is based in a principle of difference rather than of a shared rationality. As such, what is proposed here – a model of research congruent with the nomadic project which has been developed throughout this book – amounts to a fourth model of action research within the Carr and Kemmis typology.

Action research in this transgressive mood suggests three commitments: to reflexivity, collaboration and difference. The issue of reflexivity was addressed in the previous discussion of intertextuality, and is re-emphasised here in the context of the action researcher's engagement with the setting. The collaborative nature of research in this mode breaks with the traditional model of a dispassionate and detached researcher. Trangressive research practice introduces the notion that research should be constitutive of difference: that it should engage with the wider project of resistance and nomadology. Together, these commitments indicate a research which is implicitly and explicitly *engaged*· and as such must be seen as political, both at the micro-level of interpersonal power and sometimes also at the level of struggles and resistance. As such it articulates with other bodies of work which have argued for an engaged research practice, including feminist research, queer theory and disability studies.

Various writers in these areas have emphasized not only the general political commitments of research which sees itself part of the struggle to overcome oppression or inequity, but also the elision of the research/practice dualism, such that research is contiguous with and indivisible from the practical activities going on in a setting. Taking feminist approaches as an example, Ramazanoglu has argued (1992: 209) that issues such as domestic violence cannot be researched apolitically. Feminist methodologies, she suggests, have been forged not only in terms of content, but also in the context of power struggles over what it means to 'know', and what counts as valid research. Feminist commitment to resisting patriarchy has led to a suspicion of grand narratives (Holmwood 1995: 416), and a preference for research which is local, engages with the concerns of women, and values experience (Ashenden 1997, Gelsthorpe 1992: 214, Oakley 1998: 708). Oakley (1998) quotes Reinharz's (1984) comment that traditional social science research (particularly using quantitative methods) is like rape: the researchers take, hit and run.

Action research and other methodological approaches found in feminist and disability studies are thus inevitably engaged as opposed to dispassionate. They are part of a political and concomitantly an ethical project which is reflexive, collaborative and transgressive. As a footnote to this section , it is perhaps worth acknowledging that perceiving research as transgression serves as a reminder that within this model it is not possible to be restrictive as to what may or may not be undertaken as part of a 'research programme'. Rather, it is important that the open-endedness and the smoothness of the research process are acknowledged, such that any 'principles' must be constantly under review and also – as Heidegger (1958) has it – 'under erasure' as limits or striations.

Towards a Nomadology of Research

The discussions of reflexivity and intertextuality, action research and the ethico-political commitments of an engaged research suggest that a post-modern or nomadic research must reject and refuse at least the following three dualisms of

researcher vs. researched;

research vs. experience;

theory vs. practice.

I now want to set out some more considered reflections on what a nomadic approach to doing research might look like. While not intending to be prescriptive (how unnomadic that would be!), I hope these reflections will assist in both deconstructing modernist research and reconstructing something very different. The reflection will have as much to say about the epistemology and ontology, and about the implicit ethics and politics, as with details of 'how to do it'. The approach I shall adopt is to compare the nomadic and modernist perspectives at various points in the research process, picking up the three principles of postmodern research developed at the beginning of this chapter. To illustrate the points I am making, I will make reference to a research project (known as the WISDOM project) on cyber-communities and professional learning in 'virtual classrooms' in which I am involved (Fox *et al.* 1999). The salient features of the modern and postmodern approaches are summarized in Figure 7.1.

1. Setting a research question

Over a number of years spent teaching (modernist) research methods, I emphasized to students that without a clear research question it is impossible to undertake research, and that all subsequent stages in the research process are bedevilled by an absence of clarity which undermines the efforts of the researcher. However, this argument is based on the assumption that research is a linear process, and the end result of research must be some kind of 'answer' to a question. Thus a social scientist might ask the question 'how is care delivered in residential accommodation for older adults?' A natural or biomedical scientist might ask 'does ultraviolet radiation exposure lead to incidence of cutaneous melanoma in exposed subjects?' In both these questions, the outcome of the research will be judged *inter alia* upon the extent to which the research question has been answered.

	Modernist Research	Nomadic Research
The Research Question	Essential first stage in designing research	Research question must be located and related to practical issues: may take a period in the field to establish a relevant question to be asked
Research Design and Validity	Design must be adequate and appropriate. Internal validity addresses the adequacy of the design; external validity addresses the generalizability of the research	Design may require multiple methods to fully answer a question, and this will be clarified after engaging with issues in the field. Emphasis on naturalistic approaches; validity is a function of the engagement with issues relevant to the participants
Data Collection and Reliability	Data collection applies methods to minimize biases	All research entails subjective judgements, and the active engagement of the researcher is a virtue rather than a source of 'bias'
Data Analysis	The final stage of research: may enable testing of a hypothesis	Part of an on-going evaluation and reflection on the research, involving translation of findings into practical activities
Research Ethics	Weighs costs and benefits of research according to external judgements or rules	Implicit in the nomadic perspective on promoting and constituting difference and possibilities

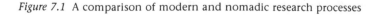

Figure 7.1 A comparison of modern and nomadic research processes

From a nomadic perspective, things are rather different. Taking the first principle of nomadic research established earlier, if *knowledge is local and contingent*, then it may not become possible to establish what are the correct questions to ask until one has a fairly clear understanding of the characteristics of the setting. A research question would only emerge after a considerable period spent familiarizing oneself with the local issues. This kind of approach to setting a research question is not wholly dissimilar to that of ethnographers and other qualitative researchers who will work in a field for an extended period, creating research questions which link to the specificities of the setting.

Taking the second principle, if the *research should be constitutive of differ- ence*, then it is important that the research question should not have the effect of closing down or limiting the ways in which the subjects of the research will be understood or will conceive of themselves. The ethics and politics of the research thus begin with the question which is asked – indeed, the concept of a 'subject' of research must be challenged and deconstructed in the research process. Within research conducted from this kind of perspective, 'subjects' become 'participants', and are not 'subjected' to research or to the will of the researcher.

Thus it will be important to involve these in the process of setting a research question which is both relevant to their own concerns and will open up rather than close down the possibilities of action available to the participants. Note that this analysis is not only applicable to social science settings in which the subjects are human, but also to natural or biomed- ical research (for example, research into human diseases or nutrition). Even if the research substrate is a cell line or an infection agent, the 'subjects' may be considered to include the human beings who will ulti- mately benefit or suffer as a consequence of the research.

The final principle, that *theory should be related to practice*, means that research questions should be developed in such a way that the theoretical consequences will be of direct practical relevance. This does not rule out 'blue sky' or 'pure' research, but does mean that researchers involved in these areas need to think carefully about the application of their research findings over a longer time period than the single investigation which they are undertaking.

To give an example of a research question which meets these criteria, in the case of the research into the potential of using computer-mediated communication for professional learning (Fox *et al.* 1999), the key research question has only finally emerged two years into the programme. It has taken that long to understand the issues, and exploratory work has been diffuse and concerned with grasping what is specific to the particular setting of a classroom established using Internet technologies. After many interviews, discussions and workshops, we now have a firm research question which addresses the processes involved in continuing professional development using networked virtual classrooms. To the extent that we worked with health professionals to establish the question, they now 'own' it, and the question articulates with their concerns and with the possibilities which might be opened up for them in the future. Concomitantly, any theory which is developed relates directly to the concerns of those involved in continuing professional development. This 'grounding' of theory is not an attempt to attain internal validity in the traditional sense in which this concept has been developed in naturalistic enquiry (Lincoln and Guba 1985), but simply to ensure that the findings are immediately relevant and setting-specific.

2. Research design, study and instrument validity

In modernist research, the issue of research design and the validity of the study and the instruments used are all tied up with the issues of whether they are appropriate and adequate to answer the research question (Cain and Finch 1981). Thus a randomized controlled trial would not be considered appropriate to answer an exploratory question of a 'how' type. Similarly a survey would not be appropriate or adequate to compare two alternative forms of treatment. In the nomadic approach, these 'technical' questions are subsumed within epistemological, political and ethical principles developed earlier.

First, if knowledge is local and contingent, we can make no assumptions about the methodological approach or the tools or instruments which should be used to uncover this 'knowledge'. Similarly, we cannot assume that one research design or instrument will be sufficient to answer a question – methodological pluralism or eclecticism may well be the key here. Just as it was necessary to spend some time in exploration before setting a research question, it will also be necessary to explore the setting fully to have a sense of how research might be pursued.

This relates to the second principle of nomadic research, in that this period of exploration should be conducted with the full involvement of all those concerned with the research, and specifically the 'subjects' or participants, as in action research designs. Conversely, the politics and ethics of difference militate against such designs as randomized and blind studies or surveys, which sustain differences between 'researcher' and the 'researched'. Methodologies which would fit into this principle include qualitative approaches which enable participation such as interviews, focus, Delphi groups and other discursive fora, case studies which are concerned with specific settings, and small- rather than large-scale approaches.

The use of such methods would also support the final principle, inasmuch as the theory which is developed from the research would be closely linked to the practical concerns of the participants, as opposed to the concerns of a 'disinterested' researcher or scientific community. As was noted in the introduction to this chapter, the difference between modernist and postmodern or nomadic research can be seen clearly in relation to issues of internal and external validity of a study. In a traditional sense, if a study concerns itself with the development of contingent and local knowledge through methods which ensure participation and the involvement of all those in a setting, then the internal validity (the extent to which a study measures what it sets out to measure) will be high. On the other hand, the external validity or generalizability to other settings will be low or non-existent. Measurements of internal and external validity would be more valuable as indicators that one's approach fits within the nomadic principles rather than as ends in themselves!

A good example of this kind of approach to research design may be found once again in the educational research on the use of 'virtual' class-rooms established using networked computers to deliver education to health professionals (Fox *et al.* 1999). The research design appropriate to a question concerning experiences of such virtual education would need to be cognisant of the particular settings (economic, cultural, religious, national etc.) in which the health professionals were located. It would be developed in conjunction with the 'learners' themselves, and would be capable of developing theory which would be relevant to the people involved in the study and relate to their own practical concerns. The design of the research has developed over a two-year period as the researchers learnt more about the setting, and the participants have been closely involved in the development of the educational programmes, and in some instances have crossed the traditional divide from 'researched' to 'researchers' themselves. In addition to collaborative educational evaluations, we are also now using Delphi approaches to draw on participants' local knowledge, to ensure relevance and utility of findings.

3. Data collection and reliability

In the traditional paradigm of modernist research, validity and reliability are closely related, with both contributing to the accuracy of the data. While validity is affected by systematic error, and is a consequence of the instrumentation or procedures developed for data collection, reliability is concerned with random error. Thus reliability is affected not so much by the adequacy of the instruments used to collect the data, but by the processes of data collection themselves. This is of great importance in social science research, where the 'instruments' may be human beings' own perceptions of situations or may involve direct interaction with subjects, for instance during interviews. Reliability may be reduced where, for example, a researcher varies the questions asked depending upon the identity or characteristics of the interviewee. Alternatively, some feature of the researcher may affect the responses made by interviewees. The 'Hawthorne' effect of enhanced performance under observation is a good example of how the data collection process may influence responses.

If the principles of nomadic research were applied to the process of data collection, from a modernist standpoint the reliability of the data would be seriously compromised, as should be obvious bearing in mind the previous discussion of design and validity. There is a requirement for a degree of reflexivity within the nomadic research process which would mean that the process of data collection would be prone to both inter- and intra-observer biases. For example, it is probable that an instrument such as a questionnaire or interview schedule would be developed in close consultation with the people who would eventually be the respondents. Indeed, the conflation of the identities of 'researcher' and 'researched' would make the concept of 'observer bias' deeply problematic.

However, rather than confounding the research process, within the nomadic paradigm, the 'bias' would be seen as a virtue, guaranteeing that the research was relevant and adequate to answer the research question. While this way of thinking about data collection is highly appropriate for social science, it might also be considered appropriate in biomedical research. For example, a research study could be devised to explore the effects of a particular drug upon patients suffering from some condition. The design of the study would involve the patients, so they would identify the parameters which were relevant for them in assessing the utility of the drug for them. These would vary from 'hard' measures of efficacy, through to the acceptability of the drug for individual patients. From a scientific perspective, the results might be seen as highly subjective, subject to random errors (loss of reliability). Within the nomadic perspective, given the reservations commented upon earlier concerning internal and external validity, the subjectivity and biases would be seen as advantages, ensuring that the research findings were relevant to the study population.

I confronted these issues when developing the research on virtual classrooms. The action research framework was highly reflexive, and participants were directly involved in the development programmes. This tended to raise issues of bias which from a modernist perspective could be seen as compromising the measurements of hard outcomes from the educational intervention. However, from an educational point of view, the research and evaluation activities were intimately tied up with the learning process outcomes, and the research instruments such as interviews often contributed to reflexivity among participants about their learning. Thus, for example, interviewing participants in the virtual classroom about their learning outcomes contributed to enhancing these outcomes.

4. Data analysis and hypothesis testing

In the modernist paradigm, the phase of data analysis completes the cycle of the research process, and should enable the research question to be answered. Where there is a hypothesis, this can be tested using inferential statistics or methods such as analytic induction (Mitchell 1983). The nomadic perspective is more open-ended than this linear or cyclical model of research. Just as the research question emerged during a preliminary exploration of the research setting, the 'analysis' of the research data is likely to be part of an on-going process of evaluation and reflection.

In terms of the first principle of nomadic research, that knowledge is local, the analysis of the data will be intimately linked with the reflections on the research process by the participants and researchers. Indeed, the 'data' would include these processes of reflection, and it would be impossible to fully understand the data if the context were to be lost or ignored (Mauthner *et al.* 1998). The second principle, that all action should be constitutive of difference, requires that the analysis of the data from the research would be constituted within the ethical and political commitments of the participants. Finally, the principle that theory should be related to practice would require that data analysis would inform the practical concerns of participants and researchers, for example through recommendations for changes in practice.

The data analysis phase is also implicated in the more general issue of the translation of research findings into practice with which I began this chapter. For these reasons, it is hard to see a clear end-point to the research process within this paradigm. There would be a blurring of the phase of 'research' with that of 'normal activity' such that in effect it is impossible to discern where one begins and the other finishes. It should be obvious from the assessment of this phase of the research process that within the nomadic paradigm, 'research' cannot be seen as an independent activity, but must be seen within the on-going ethical and political engagements of all the participants: both researchers and researched. I shall consider the translation of research findings into practice more fully in the final part of this chapter.

As an example of this kind of approach to data analysis, during the research on virtual classrooms in professional learning we have been keen to establish a rolling programme of development interventions and research. The elision of the research/practice divide was reflected in a number of aspects of the way the research was conducted:

(a) the discussions in the virtual classroom were both the material for the learning process and the successful outcome of the development programme and the data for evaluation and research;

(b) the facilitator's own involvement became part of the research 'data' and the medium of the classroom was used to encourage reflection by participants on the learning process (for a discussion of the epistemological nature of such data, see Fox and Roberts 1999);

(c) a finding from an early intervention created both a new 'research' agenda and the basis for a new learning development;

(d) participants 'graduated' from learners into facilitators and, in one or two cases to date, into 'researchers'.

These four aspects of the research process address many of the important issues in designing a research programme which meets the expectations established in the principles for postmodern or nomadic research. It is worth commenting, in conclusion, on one further aspect: the ethics of the research process. In the modernist perspective, ethical issues are often tagged on to a discussion of methods: the discussions of design, data collection and analysis are strangely shriven of any ethical or political context, and these have to be grafted on at a later stage. Bauman has been critical of the apolitical nature of modernist organization (Bauman 1989) which made such activities as the Nazi genocides simply another organizational problem to be solved by instrumental means. Similar criticism may be raised against many research practices which have flourished in the twentieth century, including many studies in psychology and the use of animals in experimentation. Research ethics weigh the benefits of research against the ethical principles upon which they impinge, and make judgements based on privileging ends against means. In contrast, there is no requirement for an additional section on the ethics of postmodern or nomadic research as it has been set out here, because the ethics and politics are totally integrated within the principles and practices of research in this paradigm. A commitment to difference (as operationalized in the emphases on reflexivity, collaboration and transgression) is in itself ethical and political. The research process flows *from* these principles, rather than remaining separate and unengaged.

Making the Difference: from Research Evidence to Practice

I began this chapter with the assertion that my agenda was a practical one, and in the following sections I have sketched out a practice-oriented nomadic model of research. I have also acknowledged that there is not a single way of doing nomadic research, but I have asserted some ethical and political principles which I believe are congruent with the nomadology I have developed in this book. So is it just a matter of choice which kind of research should be undertaken? Is it down to personal preference whether traditional methods are replaced with the kind of research process suggested here? I have argued that postmodern research brings an ethical and political dimension to the heart of doing research, and in this final section I shall argue that it does make a difference in another sense. I want to consider the relationship between research and practice from a slightly different angle: considering how research informs practice and whether a nomadic research which is integral to practice resolves some of the problems of translation which have beset modernist research. Finally, I will say a few words about the contribution that nomadic research can make to the project of nomadic embodiment and a move beyond health, setting the scene for my concluding chapter.

As I suggested earlier, there is sometimes an assumption that research ends when the paper has been published and the subjects have all – metaphorically and literally – gone home. In the model of evidence-based practice developed by writers such as Sackett *et al.* (1996), the cycle moves from question to research project to findings to review. The application of the research in practice is seen as non-problematic, something which naturally flows from the conclusions of the research. That this is actually contrary to what happens – that the uptake of research findings is actually extremely patchy – is something which has only just begun to exercise the scientific community (Dawson 1995). However, the failure to adopt research has been the subject of some interesting sociological studies, which – perhaps significantly – used ethnographic methods to explore the application of research.

Callon (1986) has told an entertaining tale of what happened when some scientists sought to influence the practice of fisher-folk in France. With a crisis in the scallop industry resulting from over-fishing, laboratory reports of methods to farm these molluscs were bound to be important.

The first problem arose when it was found that scallops which grew successfully in the laboratory setting would not attach themselves to rocks in the sea. Two years of field-work appeared to resolve the problem, but the project required co-operation from the fishing community to allow the new colony to become established. Disagreements between the fisher-folk and the marine biologists concerning the important issues left an uneasy peace, and with quotas seriously reduced, the fishing community was disaffected with the scientists, whose intervention had reduced their incomes. A final dispute led to a midnight orgy of over-fishing in the new scallop community, which left the scientific project in ruins, but ensured the fishing community a happy Christmas on the proceeds of their one-off catch! Callon concluded that the fishers and biologists had such divergent perspectives that it was impossible to translate the scientific arguments into a form which seemed relevant to the people who depended on the scallops for their livelihood.

In the context of health care, Wood *et al.* (1998) asked why it was that some initiatives based on research evidence were translated into practice, while others were unsuccessful in overcoming established but evidentially unsubstantiated practice. They looked at evidence-based guidelines on such issues as the use of oral anticoagulants for stroke prophylaxis, laparoscopic surgery for inguinal hernia repair and the proposals for obstetric care set out in a government circular known as 'Changing Childbirth'. While there appeared to be general acceptance of the last, other initiatives were often adopted patchily, and in the case of anticoagulant prophylaxis, there was very slow implementation despite the evidence of reduced morbidity and mortality. Wood *et al.* suggest that practitioners are not convinced by disembodied research findings, but want to see these findings contextualized within their own practical experience (1998: 1734).

> In promoting an innovation or piece of research we are not dealing with the uncomplicated dissemination of findings to a largely passive and receptive audience – a simple problem of 'putting theory *into* practice' in the hackneyed sense of the phrase – but with the question of reconnecting research with its supplementary other: practice. (ibid.: their emphasis)

They found it essential that practitioners 'bought in' to the proposed changes, and that research had to take account of locally situated practices which engage with the research. They argue that for research to be implemented required a willingness to see things from a range of perspectives, and to acknowledge that any 'research findings' represent not so much truth about reality, as a reified moment in an on-going and indeterminate process (ibid.: 1735).

Research and practice need to be seen as differing world-views on the same subject matter: researchers see data while practitioners (hopefully) see people (Haines and Jones 1994). Research data must be translated from the former to the latter world-view before it is recognized as relevant by practitioners. Shaugnessy *et al.* (1994) suggest that the perceived utility of evidence by practitioners will depend on its relevance to a particular setting, and its validity for that setting. Studies conducted in one setting may not easily transfer to another, and practitioners need to recognize a problem for which the evidence is relevant, before research will be seen as applicable in a practice setting (Williamson 1992).

Research evidence is most likely to be adopted by practitioners if it is first 'digested' or synthesized, replacing specific findings (the usual outcome of a particular study), with a 'big picture'. For instance, guidelines for health-care practice integrate research into the wider social and cultural circumstances in which practical care is undertaken (Brown and Duguid 1991, Haynes 1993). Such guidelines work best if they are produced locally and as part of a bottom-up approach to implementation (Grimshaw and Russell 1993, Haines and Jones 1994).

There are strong arguments here for the research process, not the least of which is that when planning dissemination of research findings, researchers must abandon any arrogance concerning the subsequent use of the findings. Instead, research findings need to engage with the practice that they wish to inform. I would argue that the nomadic model set out in this chapter is one way of assuring that findings are seen as useful, relevant and valid, by removing the barriers between and dichotomies of researcher/researched, research/experience and theory/practice. Nomadic research has value only in its application, and existence only in engaged, reflexive and participative settings.

A Final Reflection on Research and Practice

I have set out a detailed programme for a nomadologically-informed approach to research in this chapter, and made some highly critical comments about the failures of modernist research. For two reasons, I do not wish to argue that the approach developed here is exclusively the 'best' way to do research.

First, as noted earlier, if the research process is intrinsically transgressive, that rules out there being a single truth about how things should be done. Indeed, reflexivity about practice requires that one is always critical and open to new ways of thinking. Nomadology is about taking a situation and 'thinking upside-down' (Handy 1991), recognizing possibilities and novelty. So it is not the case that all research must conform to one way of doing things: rather, there may be merits in a wide variety of approaches. But I would contend that researchers need to reflect upon their methods and think about those dualisms which I mentioned a moment ago, to consider their engagement with the world they purport to describe and explain. Watson *et al.* (1995) speak of methodology under erasure, adopting the Heideggerian and Derridean technique of using a word and acknowledging its inadequacy to signify. In a different sense, I suggest that 'methodology under erasure' reminds us that we cannot achieve unmediated knowledge of the world, and that unless we engage with the world reflexively, any methodology is nothing more than a conceit.

Second, and of less consequence, is the question of the 'validity' of the data which I have used elsewhere in this text and in other writings. Neither my work on surgery nor the later studies of care fully meet the criteria set out here, yet I have used this 'data' to develop arguments for nomadology! Readers are of course entitled to see this as a fatal logical flaw (though, heck – Garfinkel (1967) did it when he undermined the interpretations which he had earlier used to develop his propositions concerning ethnomethodology, so why shouldn't I?). On the other hand, these diverse methodological approaches can be seen as nomadic wanderings, meandering towards, around and away from 'truth', but still offering up 'truths' which can evoke (Tyler 1986), deterritorialize and transgress when taken as part of a reflexive and engaged project.

I hope this chapter has done more than simply set out a rival model of research. The ideas developed here have much to say to the academic or the contract researcher, but also to those engaged in practice. I have tried to show that research can be seen as integral to practice, as 'everybody's business'. Further, I would suggest that the principles for nomadic research – of knowledge being contingent, of being always on the side of difference, and of being fully engaged – are implicated throughout practice. In common with my thoughts on risk, there is an ethics and a politics here which have much to say to those who engage with issues of embodiment, whether as care practitioners or in everyday personal engagements.

8
Lines of Flight

The Beyond

Imagine a surface – the top of a table, for instance – which is deeply rutted. Imagine yourself as a billiard ball, lying in one of those ruts. How do you feel? Trapped? Stuck in a rut? However much you want it, you cannot raise yourself high enough even to flip over into the next rut. Now imagine that the tabletop is being slowly tipped up from its horizontal position. At some point, depending on how deep the ruts are, the billiard ball *does* flip over the lip of the rut into the next one along. If the table is tipped sufficiently, the ball doesn't simply flip over, but carries on, bouncing along the tops of the ruts, landing in a rut but with enough momentum to flip right out again.

If you feel you are in a rut, or trapped by what's going on in your life – money, relationships, a routine job, the ritual of ever-repeated everyday activities – maybe what is needed is to tip the table. Tip it a little and you'll flip over: okay, so you're in a rut again, but at least it's a different rut. Tip it more, and you'll bounce over the ruts and end up who knows where.

Tipping the table (changing the force of gravity that gives the ruts their 'stickiness') is a way of creating what Deleuze and Guattari call a *line of flight* out of territory. If you (your body) is becoming-other, it is on a line of flight, defined by movement and rest (Deleuze and Guattari 1988: 276). It cannot be *pinned down*, it slips in everywhere, it is constantly in flux. The being-body on the other hand has had its movement stolen from it, it is territorialized, held firmly in place. In the first chapters of the book, I suggested some ways this happens, as frames of time, space, care, professionalism are applied to the body to steal its movement away. In subsequent chapters I have suggested how these frames can be resisted and overthrown. To resist is to forge a line of flight.

A moment for exegesis. Deterritorialization is the movement by which a body leaves a territory, and is the operation of a line of flight (Deleuze and Guattari 1988: 508). The line of flight may lead in any direction: all we know is that it leads us away. The deterritorialization may be overlaid with a compensatory reterritorialization which obstructs the line of flight, in which case the deterritorialization is negative, it leads directly into some new territory, a new rut (and a new Body-without-Organs). Or relative deterritorialization, which – although it overwhelms the reterritorializations – has a line of fight which is segmented, which is drawn into new spaces along the way, each with its own vectors, territorializations and deterritorializations (which lead into the known). Or absolute deterritorialization, built upon relative deterritorialization, which is that movement which finally breaks away, achieves escape velocity to create a new space and connect lines of flight creatively in a blitzkrieg that ensures there is no falling back into a new territory (Deleuze and Guattari 1988: 508–10).

The last two chapters have given examples of what may happen to lines of flight. For the surgeon or the clubber whose life-choices are trammelled by the fear-mongering pundits of risk assessment, their lines of flight lead to negative deterritorialization as stigmatized risk-takers. Alternatively, if these choices are seen as just that, parts of an unfolding life course, the line of flight enables a relative deterritorialization, opening up new possibilities for action, new territories to inhabit and perhaps to move beyond, even into an absolute deterritorialization. For participants in a research project, a traditional researcher/researched dualism carries them straight to a reterritorialization as 'subjects', disempowered and disengaged. Those involved in transgressive action research find a line of flight which can lead to new ways of understanding themselves and their environment, new possibilities to know and to challenge other truths.

This book can be a line of flight; it is certainly about the line of flight which can lead *beyond health*. This idea of the *beyond*, which is so redolent of transcendence, is not transcendent at all (Deleuze and Guattari 1988: 510); rather it is about connecting lines of flight, turning negative deterritorialization to relative deterritorialization to absolute deterritorialization. The test of this book's line of flight comes after you put it down. Is this physically final chapter also the final moment before a reterritorialization which leads back to control and subjugation as you turn back to familiar territory, or the jumping-off point which takes you to unknown territories, to become the nomad inhabitant of smoother spaces?

The test of any line of flight is the same: the proof is in the pudding, so to speak. You won't know the outcome until you try; you can't move beyond health unless you choose to do exactly that, and even then there is no guarantee of success. Because these lines of flight are everywhere, and have been conjugated into such a tangled web, many have been short-circuited to lead straight back into what has – variously throughout this book – been called territory, regimes of truth or the frames which constitute and mediate power and control. But these conjunctions are continually unravelling, releasing lines of flight which make resistance possible, and open the way to smoother spaces and nomadic subjectivity. To maximize the lines of flight, this final chapter approaches health and embodiment from a variety of angles, to increase the vectors (directions and velocity), to unravel the web: to turn a text into a practical exercise in nomadology.

In Search of Smoother Space

I used the metaphor of a rutted tabletop to imagine territorialization; Deleuze and Guattari speak of *striated space*, the same notion. If these striations could be stretched out, pulled taut like the smoothing of a crumpled tablecloth, the result would be similar: the ruts would disappear, we would have *smooth space* instead. Striated and smooth spaces have different relations to motion – Deleuze and Guattari make connections with the *nomad* and nomadic relations with the land they pass through.

> In striated space, lines or trajectories tend to be subordinated to points: one goes from one point to another. In the smooth, it is the opposite: the points are subordinated to the trajectory. This was already the case among the nomads for the clothes–tent–space vector of the outside. The dwelling is subordinated to the journey; inner space conforms to outside space: tent, igloo, boat. There are stops and trajectories in both the smooth and the striated. But in smooth space, the stop follows from the trajectory. (Deleuze and Guattari 1988: 478)

We know a lot (unless we are nomads) about striated space, because for most of us that is where we live our lives. It is filled with things, formed into recognizable identities which constitute an irreducible materiality: matter. It is the space of organization, measurement and attributes (Deleuze and Guattari 1988: 479). In striated space, we are this, or this, or whatever we have found ourselves to be. Bodies have organs, they are circumscribed, solid, unchanging. We are defined into existence until there is no room for doubt or alternative. It is the space of the realist, whose perceptions are so much part of constituting the reality, whose outlook confirms and reifies the confines of this space.

Smooth space is perceived less in terms of dimensions and places, as in directions. It is filled with events rather than with 'things'; it is a space of affects (or relations) rather than properties or attributes. Smooth space is occupied by intensities: 'wind and noise, forces, and sonorous and tactile qualities, as in the desert, steppe or ice. The creaking of ice and the song of the sands' (ibid). Bodies are without organs, they are becoming rather than being, as their intensities vary along lines of flight. There is no sense of departure or arrival, of beginning or end, only of travelling, of being in motion. Yet one cannot be lost in smooth space, because that would imply that there is something which might be found, a purpose, objective or right place to be. In smooth space, everywhere is as 'right' as everywhere else.

Have you found a smooth space? Perhaps it was during travel, a moment when the motion of your body became all that there was. Not because you did not want to reach your destination, just that travelling, the sheer sense of movement, came to be all that was required. Or perhaps it was some other beyond, a moment of dissolution, of laughter, orgasm, spiritual ecstasy or even pain. In that moment or minute or hour or day, the ruts were pulled taut, your subjectivity was free to roam across the steppes of the soul, into smooth space.

In smooth space there is no need to be one thing, to sustain a fixed identity. You can be whatever you wish, what is important is not who you are, or who or what else there is in smooth space. There is no longer a 'you' or a 'me' anyway, or trees or parents or governments for that matter, there are only *events* or what Deleuze and Guattari (1988: 261) call *haecceities*. A haecceity has two components. First, its relations of movement or rest – its *longitude*; second, the affects or relations (I will say more about these in the next section) of which it is capable – its *latitude* (ibid.: 260).

To find a line of flight into smooth space requires only (but it is a very big 'only') a realization that a body is merely longitude and latitude, movements and affects:

> a set of speeds and slownesses between unformed particles, a set of nonsubjectified affects. You have the individuality of a day, a season, a year, a *life* (regardless of its duration) – a climate, a wind, a fog, a swarm, a pack (regardless of its regularity). Or at least you can have, you can reach it. ... It is the wolf itself, and the horse, and the child, that cease to be subjects to become events, in assemblages that are inseparable from an hour, a season, an atmosphere, an air, a life. The street enters into composition with the horse, just as the dying rat enters into composition with the air, and the beast and the full moon enter into composition with each other. (Deleuze and Guattari 1988: 262)

Once in smooth space, there is no longer subject, no longer identity, only patterns of intensity, marked out on a plane of pure difference. Because in smooth space, a haecceity *is* the relations and affects which connect bodies, the body cannot be separated from other haecceities.

> Climate, wind, season, hour are not of another nature than the things, animals, people that populate them, follow them, sleep and awaken within them. This should be read without a pause: the animal-stalks-at-five-o'clock. The becoming evening, becoming-night of an animal, blood nuptials. Five o'clock is the animal! This animal is this place! ... A haecceity has neither beginning nor end, origin nor destination; it is always in the middle. It is not made of points, only of lines. (ibid.: 263)

Smooth space is what is *beyond*, not in a transcendental sense but in a material sense, if only we can break out of the striated space which creates us as identities, selves, bodies subjected by force and territorialized into bodies-with-organs. Lines of flight lead *beyond*, into the deterritorialized nomadism of a space populated by haecceities possessing only speed and affect, longitude and latitude. We were there at least once before, and it is possible to get back there again.

We have been led into striated space since our socialization into culture began. We are told 'don't do that' or 'do this'; 'don't behave like that, be like this' (Deleuze and Guattari 1988: 276). We are inscribed into our culture's idea of a human, or a woman or a black or a patient; we are disciplined till we accept striated space as the only one there is. Striated space is not a good place to be, it is not the safe haven some might believe. It is fraught, because the relations we establish as we inhabit striated space can lead to some very bad things indeed.

What Can a Body Do?

In an essay which focuses attention on a key element in Deleuze and Guattari's ontology, Buchanan suggests that theorists of the body (in philosophy, social science and biomedicine) have been asking the wrong question. Rather than considering what a body *is*, they should ask: *what can a body do?* This question

> is the critical means of finding out what masochists, drug users, obsessives and paranoiacs are actually trying to do. The question works by staking out an area of *what* a body actually can do. This area is restricted by obvious physical constraints which must be respected. But this does

not mean that there is no beyond, or that a beyond cannot be desired. And it is just this *beyond* – beyond the physical limits of the physical body – that the concept of the body-without-organs articulates. ... It is the body's limits that define the BwO, not the other way around. (Buchanan 1997: 79, his emphases)

By asking this question, we abandon efforts to define the essential nature of a body. Yet this is not a recourse to functionalism, because the answer to the question consists not in assessing cause/effect (it has kidneys, so it can excrete), but in counting the *affects* or *relations* of a body (Deleuze and Guattari 1988: 257), which may be many or few. Here is a question which recognizes an active, choice-making, engaged and engaging body, not one passively written in systems of thought. Bodies are not the locus at which forces act, they are the production of the interactions of forces. A body is *the capacity to form new relations, and the desire to do so* (Buchanan 1997: 83).

A body can do this and it can do that, according to its species, to the situations/settings/territories it inhabits, and to its aspirations within an unfolding, choice-making, active living. A blackbird sings *inter alia* because it has vocal chords (and neural pathways) which can form a relation with air that results in song. It has a relation to the dawning day or to predators in its environment. And the singing blackbird has serendipitous relations with other bodies (blackbirds and other animals) concerning mating, or warning, or marking territory. For human beings, things are more complicated, but the principle is the same. They have relations which are proper to their species, to their environment, and to their aspirations to talk, to work, to love, to reason or whatever.

It is the forces – of biology, of environment, of culture and reflexivity, and of the aspirational potential which all living things possess – which together make the body. They do this by defining (constraining, elaborating) the body's relations or affects: what it can do. Hence the structure of this book, documenting first the forces and the resistances, which together constitute the becoming-body (as opposed to an essentialist being-body). Asking the question of a body: what can it do? (which are its relations?) informs us about its Body-without-Organs (which are the confluences of a body with its affects – what Deleuze and Guattari call variously machines or assemblages), about territory and nomadism (the forces that make it what it is and what it may become), about deterritorialization and lines of flight (the trajectories which open up possibilities for becoming-other). For Deleuze and Guattari, this has both a theoretical significance and a practical engagement, including the creation of a basis for their 'schizoanalysis'. By encouraging patients (or people) to pursue an aspiration, it opens locked doors to new vistas (Buchanan 1997: 85). Importantly, this

> does not result in the patient being restored to his or her former self, rather, using the newly awakened affect, he or she is encouraged to invent a new self. ... [This formulation avoids] the inevitable closure of standard hermeneutic accounts of the embodied self that picture it as a mostly stable negotiation between the instinctual desires of nature and the necessary compromise of culture. (Buchanan 1997: 85–6)

Both 'natural' and 'cultural' forces comprise the relations which a body can have (and thus, what it can do), both are implicated in the 'self-invention' which is both a feature of schizoanalysis, and more generally of nomadology. Counting the relations ('natural' or 'cultural' – these terms become meaningless) of a body can indicate how it is territorialized; fostering new relations may open the way to a line of flight.

So let us ask this question about the human body. In Buchanan's essay, he focuses on some BwOs which are congruent with the Deleuze and Guattari project: the anorexic body, the paralysed body, the schizoid body (Buchanan 1997: 8ff), just as Deleuze and Guattari (1988: 150) consider the hypochondriac, drugged and masochistic bodies. I want to look at some less extreme BwOs, which may help map the limits of the *healthy* body (including its implicit antithesis, the sick body), and hence the lines of flight which might change those limits. In these sketches, think about relations/affects, about territorialization and about lines of flight.

The fit body

The body has a relation to gravity: it resists it and yet requires it for its creation and its sustenance. Gravity is an addiction, yet unlike a drug whose addict craves its ingestion, here the addiction is concerned with refusing its victory. The muscles of the body enter into new relations with the skin: pressing outwards, testing its limits. There are relations with fat and heart disease, which have become the enemy: the fit body wages poignant war on itself, denying (yet simultaneously admitting) its relation to time and to degradation.

The growing body

The body has a relation with time and with space. It aspires to have moved beyond where it is now, for time to have passed, for space to have been filled; alternatively it aspires always to remain the same, to return to what it was before. It tests its new capacities against the environment, and measures itself against what it has been, and what it will be in the future. Its relation to the environment is one of absorption, of nutrients and of experience.

The slimming body

The body enhances, concentrates and strengthens its relation with food, it thinks of everything it sees: 'I can consume you, you can become part of me.' Life is measured in kilograms and days: the body becomes utopian, Puritan and millenarian, imagining a time and a remade, slim body which has yet to come into existence but which once attained will be free of pain and longing, gloriously released from the shackles of unconsummated desire.

The shopping body

The body has a relation with absent goods; a lack of things which must be remedied as quickly and as efficiently as possible. The body's possessions have lost their lustre, its aspiration turns only towards things it does not yet possess. The shopping body is single-minded and conservative: only that to which it aspires will do. It carries its successes like designer-labelled medals.

The valetudinarian body

This body has been consumed by the diseases it fears. There is nothing left, it has been burnt out, it has become pathology. The BwO rattles, like an empty husk whose only contents are the ailments which began this dismal territorialization.

The career(ing) body

There is a relation to a future body, in which the present body imagines itself to be the future body. The future body is more-something (more rich, more secure, more socially connected and so on). This future more-body assimilates the present body, casting it in the role of precursor, cause, father or child. The future more-body establishes itself as dictator of the present body, measuring out how much the present body must do to assure its more-body.

The cancerous (cancering) body

The body subjects itself to censorship, to moralistic outrage. It appraises itself: 'this part is good, it can remain; this part is bad, it must be excised or burnt or poisoned or overcome by positive mental effort'. The body is conservative, it is suspicious of novelty, of otherness: it is a control freak because the worst consequence is to lose control.

The aroused (arousing) body

The body has a relation with its own organs of erotic sensation, which it almost always dissembles, elaborating fictions that the relation is with some one or some thing other than the body itself. The aroused body aspires to its own destruction through orgasm, yet wishes that destruction to be infinitely prolonged.

The senescent or dying body

The body has a relation to time: it passes time by giving its capacities away, until there is nothing left to give, no more aspiration. It is engaged in giving up all that was once needed, saying 'I no longer have a use for this or that, what do I want with that any more?' When the body is emptied of all it contained, it no longer aspires to anything.

And so on.

In writing these abstractions, I have tried to elaborate the ambivalence of the affects or relations, and their capacity to become all-consuming. All these bodies are active, and they are all becoming-other (the exercising body is becoming-fit, the valetudinarian body is becoming-invalid, the dying body is becoming-moribund), they all are constitutive of BwOs as they conjoin with their affects (there is a food-eating body confluence and a goods-shopping body confluence and so on). Yet becoming is risky, which is why Deleuze and Guattari warn of the hazardous business of making a BwO:

> ... you make one, you can't desire without making one. ... This is not reassuring, because you can botch it. Or it can be terrifying, and lead you to your death. (Deleuze and Guattari 1988: 149)

It is in the intensification of an affect or relation that the danger lies. Buchanan uses the example of the anorexic (the 'slimming body' gone critical, perhaps), who

> endeavours to obtain freedom, to become free, via the pathway of an intensive hunger, eliminating in the process all extensive demand (demands of the body-organism). Hunger that is not determined by the demands of the body is intense because it is now for itself; as such, it would be more correct to describe it as 'hungering' not hunger. The problem for the anorexic, however, and this is the inherent danger of all self-motivated becoming, is that far from accelerating becoming, what he or she actually does is deform it. Intensifying a particular

(affect is) ... a gross delimitation of becoming itself. It confuses the blissfully passive beyond of becoming which Nietzsche idealizes, with the passivity of the already become. (Buchanan 1997: 87)

A body (BwO) that has become (rather than in the process of becoming) is victim of a negative territorialization which leads directly into a reterritorialization, but into a territory which cannot be easily escaped: there are no longer any lines of flight. The valetudinarian has become an invalid, no more than a vehicle for her ills; the careerist has become workaholic and finds no meaning outside work; the aroused body has become attached to its object of affect and finds no pleasure in other relations. Having become, there is no becoming left to do. Seeking a line of flight, it has been led right back into deeply striated space.

Becoming requires the multiplication of affect, not the intensification of a single affect or relation. It is an opening-up to difference, to possibility and to the 'rightness' of the many rather than the few or the one. Singularity of purpose leads not to the beyond, but to death. In achieving multiplicity, we need all the help we can get.

The Ethics and Politics of Nomadology

The previous paragraphs could be read as a solipsist manifesto, in which the only reality is one's own imagination, how one 'thinks oneself'. As such, it is a kind of Buddhist exercise in meditating oneself out of material reality into nirvana (a transcendent beyond), or a Christian Scientist philosophy (Eddy 1994) of overcoming material suffering through spiritual intervention. This interpretation is incorrect for two reasons. First, because it reintroduces a mind/body division, privileging the mind as the arena of becoming and the body as mere substance to be moulded in the mind's eye. Rather, as Deleuze and Guattari conceive it, the mind and body are parts of the same materiality, in which sense-of-self or subjectivity is one consequence of the dynamics of forces and resistances. Mind (or 'minding') is an event or haecceity in the same way as are skin ('retaining') and genitalia ('sexing'). 'Selfing' is the becoming other of one kind of affect of which the human body is capable (and it is prone to the same risks as any other becoming – that it may have already become).

The second reason to reject a solipsist version of nomadology should also be clear from what has gone before, and also from this last point. It concerns the responsibility and commitment to difference, to the becoming-other body which goes to the heart of this perspective. It is because of the dangers involved in becoming (which I have indicated above in my vignettes of the becoming-bodies) that an affect or relation will overcome the BwO, filling it, excluding any other capacities, ensuring its status as already become. What if through our action (intentional or not), we should contribute to the already-become body of another? Are we to stand by, and say 'well, that's her problem or his choice'?

To answer that question, I want to recall the material I documented in the first section of the book. Remember the surgeon who constructed (framed) the patients so they left or stayed in hospital according to the surgeon's wish? Remember the carers who imposed a regime of vigilance over their charges? Remember the older adults whose lives were overwhelmed by 'empty time' and constrained by the restrictions of their living spaces?

Are these patients and people not precisely the already-become bodies which have been led into a reterritorialization from which there is no way out (or almost – there is always a way out if you can only find it)? Are not these professionals the people who have done this reterritorialization? On the other hand, what of the carers whose *gifts* were so precious to the older adults or to the others described in chapter 3? Are these not the people who are deterritorializing, enabling lines of flight, opening up possibilities for others to become and to continue becoming?

In short, everything that I have written in this book so far is part of an ethics and a politics. I have argued throughout that difference can be the basis for this ethico-political engagement. This may be in terms of how we react to people's choices (chapter 6) – celebrating difference and avoiding ascriptions of 'risk' or 'safety' to these choices. Or it could be about how we conduct research and seek knowledge about the world in which we live (chapter 7), seeking methods which are constitutive of difference and transgressive of established 'truth'. But whatever is involved, it is about an *engagement* with the world, not a *disengagement*. Nomadology cannot be simply about rethinking our own private worlds and our own bodies. Apart from anything else – unless we chance upon it, or maybe have the qualities (affects) of a Gandhi or a Jesus of Nazareth – the line of flight which will enable nomadism will probably remain elusive. Which of us, after all, can resist the reterritorializing force of the 'diseasing' (cancering, stroking, dementing) body? (Deleuze, maybe, who leapt from an upstairs window to his death?)

The ethics and politics of nomadology and the line of flight celebrate difference and multiplicity of affect, and avoid definition and identity. As such they have something in common with some other efforts to develop a postmodern ethics. For example, Bauman, following Levinas, argues that proximity to others (faciality) and a willingness to open oneself to the Other constitutes a basis for an ethical subject. We are responsible for facing and embracing otherness, while constraining our own behaviour (Bauman 1993b: 74, 220). Caputo argues for a postmodern minimalism concerning moral codes: responsibilities to others, he says 'happen', they are local affairs, matters of flesh and blood (Caputo 1993: 227). From the different perspective of communitarianism, Etzioni argues that the highly differentiated human societies of the modern period bring responsibilities linked to the rights which are claimed for human beings (Etzioni 1995: 10). Difference can be associated with the principle of solidarity, argues Leonard (1997: 164), to underpin a postmodern ethic.

In my own view, it is the association of the *celebration of difference* with an emphasis on *engagement* with the world that provides nomadology with its practical and ethico-political edge, and it is in a focus on practice that the ethico-political agenda is spelt out. To put it another way, the question 'What can a body do?' is not so much an academic query as a rallying cry. As we engage with others, we may ask of them, and of ourselves 'What can this body – in front of me right now – do?'

Throughout this book I have drawn on the work of White (1991) as suggesting an engagement with the world in a spirit of a celebration of difference. White argues for an engaged response that is quite different from a modernist engagement grounded in a *will to mastery* and a *perceived responsibility to act*. (This latter may be seen in theories and codes of professional conduct which encourage active engagement – potentially regardless of outcome or impact, or research which is grounded in the premise that the end justifies the means.) White posits an alternative ethical engagement based in a *responsibility to otherness*. This is the rejection of a will to mastery, and the substitution of this *proper*, identity-seeking discourse with a *gift* relation, in which that which is other, different and diverse is celebrated. White suggests that the 'mood' of such an engagement based in a *gift* might be one of 'grieving delight'. This mood would

> come alive in the spacing between the self and otherness. The delight with the appearance of the other brings with it the urge to draw it closer. But that urge must realise its limits, beyond which the drawing nearer becomes a gesture of grasping. And that realisation will be palpable only when we are sensitive to the appearance of the particular other as testimony of finitude. (White 1991: 90)

With such a perspective, it is much more likely that our engagement will be sustained on the side of difference, that it will foster lines of flight rather than reterritorialization. We are sensitized to the injustices of force, while the delight in difference deepens a commitment to becoming-other. This 'nomadic sensibility' can never be disengaged: indeed it is always seeking closer and more profound engagement.

This ethico-political dimension to nomadology translates into the realization that *embodiment must be understood as an unfinished project.* The body is not a biological entity, nor is it a cultural artefact; rather, it is an unfolding process ('bodying' if you will), in which nature and culture are aspects of a panoply of forces and resistances. Embodiment is process: the living, growing becoming which is always in flux. Nomadology is not an add-on: it is a reminder of this processual quality to embodiment, a tool for its enhancement, and an admonition for those who would – through force, definition or essentialist doctrine – fix or limit the body.

The body lives, therefore it is nomadic! All we need do is recognize this, and use this realization in our engagements. This holds for human engagement in general, but also for those specific engagements (which may extend from the caresses of a lover to the tending to the sick or dying) which we call care.

Questions for Health Professionals and People with Bodies

Together, the formulations of nomadology developed in this chapter and the ethico-political engagement around a responsibility to otherness constitute a radically different conception of human potential (what has traditionally been so narrowly defined as 'health') and of what constitutes the 'care' which engages with this potential. Health is the becoming-other of haecceities or body-affect confluences in lines of flight. The objective of care in this perspective is about enhancing or facilitating these becoming and possibilities, about resistance to force, and a generosity towards otherness. It is a process which offers promise, rather than fulfilling it, offers possibility in place of certainty, multiplicity in place of repetition, difference in place of identity (Fox 1993a: 160). It is the *gift* which expects no recognition.

In chapter 3, I suggested that care was paradoxical, and I outlined the conflicts between the two irreconcilable elements of care, as *vigil* and as *gift*. This paradox is not abstract, it is a practical issue which challenges carers as they evaluate and valorize their activities.

It cannot be readily resolved without the kind of analysis which has been suggested in this chapter concerning bodies and their relations (what a body can – or might – do), lines of flight and deterritorialization. Modernism offers nothing other than a responsibility to act, and no vantage point from which to discern and evaluate the consequences of this action before it may be too late. Carers decide: 'yes we must act to sustain our patients emotionally or spiritually', yet this decision is taken knowing little or nothing about what that means for the others of care themselves, in their specific situations or with their particular body-affect confluences.

The promise of postmodernism and nomadology for our engagements (those which we call 'caring' and other relations our bodies make) is to re-engage not with categories or types, but with individuals marked out by their differences, not what they have in common. It forces us to reflect upon what it is to be human, and to engage with other human beings. There is no longer a simple recipe for a caring (or other engagement) which enables; no formula can provide the answer.

But all the words in this book have been written to show how a non-essentialist resisting subject can be modelled, and how this can provide some cues to practice. In this chapter I outlined two elements constitutive of nomadology: a celebration of difference and a commitment to engagement. It could also be considered in terms of the three principles developed in the last chapter: that knowledge is local and contingent, that action should be constitutive of difference, and that knowledge should be oriented towards practice (in the widest sense of what happens, what bodies do). Either way, some pertinent questions can be suggested, both for care professionals as they address issues of 'health', and more generally, for people with bodies. These and the meditation which follows, replace any neat formula for how to care, or how to engage. The questions may be asked both in terms of an ethics and politics of engagement, and in terms of one's own becoming-other.

1. When you engage with the world (that is, when your body makes a relation with some aspect of the world), are you on the side of the nomad thought? Do you delight in the wandering nomad broken free (for however short a time) from a territory? From such a position comes the reflection that engagement is to be judged in terms of its consequences for others (and otherness), not by any overarching discourse of good or truth.

2. If you have values, are these grounded in a celebration of difference and otherness? Are your values flexible enough to avoid the structures, systems and repetitions which force us into sameness? Recognize the undecidability and openness of the world, its capacity always to become other.

3. When you desire something (engage with it), do you desire (engage) in a spirit of generosity, not to attain mastery or control over it? Do not try to possess the object of your desire (the *other*); make it possible that your relation to it is a gift requiring no response or repetition.

4. When you are offered a gift (knowingly or unknowingly) by another, do you take pleasure in it or see it as something which must be reciprocated? Open yourself to the gifts which can deterritorialize your body.

5. What can your body do (what are the sum of its relations)? Can it do more now than it could in the past, or less? If the answer is less, start over with these questions.

A Meditation on the Nomad

This meditation is based upon a reflection on infinite friendliness. It can be adapted to focus on the areas of affect which are the most resistant to nomad subjectivity. Note that the purpose is not to disengage you from what you love or enjoy, but *to re-engage* you with things for which you have little or no time.

Think about a place that you feel really happy in. It could be your home, or a place you have visited. Think about all the feelings which are associated with this location, what it means to you, and what makes this place so special (5 minutes).

Now think about a place which you really dislike, which makes you feel uncomfortable or to which you have other strong negative feelings. Also think about somewhere that you feel indifferent towards: which has neither the positive nor the negative aspects which you have previously identified. Try to select places that are currently part of your life rather than distant in time or space (5 minutes).

Now bring the three places together in your thoughts. Try to respond to the places you dislike or towards which you are indifferent in the same way that you feel about the 'good place'. It may be very hard to begin with for you to do this with the location you dislike. If so, focus on the place which has no significance either way. Allow your response to change, so that now you feel about the places the same way, no longer privileging the 'good' place over the other. Allow yourself to respond as positively to the indifferent location and eventually – if you can – to the place you initially disliked as you feel towards your 'good place' (5 minutes).

Finally, put your positive attitude to work in a *practical* way: re-engage in some way in your life with these previously rejected or negative places.

(Note, this does not mean you have to go and hang out in a dangerous neighbourhood at 2 a.m.! But it could mean doing something to try to make this place less dangerous.)

On another occasion, do the same for another aspect of your life which is important to you. For example:

A good friend – someone you have no feelings towards either way – someone you dislike;

An aspect of your job or studies which you like – an aspect towards which you are indifferent – something you don't like about the work;

Something in your life or the way you are about which you are happy and pleased – something which does not matter either way – something about your life or yourself you do not like or want to change.

In each case, the objective is to foster a confluence of affect and body (place–moving body, job–working body) which is open to possibilities rather than closed into an opposition or polarization of good vs. bad, wanted vs. not wanted.

In Pursuit of the Nomad: the Personal and the Political

I want to end with a short reflection on what the ideas developed in this book, and in particular in this final chapter, mean for me. When I completed writing my last book in 1993, I had little idea of the ways that work would impact on my life. *Postmodernism, Sociology and Health* (Fox 1993a) had been in my head for at least five years, and a thesis and a book-of-the-thesis had to come first. While its publication consequently felt like the fulfilment of a long-held ambition, because the text had seemed to gain a life of its own during the writing, the book still seemed fresh and satisfying when it appeared.

But writing *Postmodernism, Sociology and Health* forced me to challenge just about every basis for personal meaning that I had, because of its unremitting rejection of the meta-narratives of modernity. Had I been fully up to speed with Deleuze and Guattari's theoretical framework at that point, I would have said that I was ripe for nomadism. I had been deterritorialized, and was on a line of flight which led me subsequently in some unexpected directions. One of these was an unsolicited discovery of a spirituality after a life as an atheist, which at least in its atavistic form was something of an embarrassment for a self-proclaimed postmodernist! But the central message of Christianity concerning love, particularly as refracted through the postmodern lens of such works as Stephen Mitchell's (1991) *The Gospel According to Jesus* and Don Cupitt's (1994) *After All*, helped me to develop concepts such as the *gift* which I had written about. This led me both into new places and into the company of people with whom I had previously had no contact, and into an interest in care.

This latter interest in turn took me in 1997 to Thailand and Australia to do the field-work on older adults' experiences of care which has been reported in this book. Both the experience of being a lone traveller for an extended period, and the opportunity to do a piece of cross-cultural work contributed further to the 'nomadic' streak in my new persona. The otherness of south-east Asia (once off the tourist track) and the sheer size and alienness of Australia gave me a sense of what it meant to become-other, to lose oneself in the geographical and philosophical by-ways of the world. My fascination with Australia has become a love affair, with two subsequent trips and more planned for the future. Its size and emptiness, as well as its original inhabitants' lifestyle, make it a place for me in which the nomadic is manifest.

Travelling is good for practising nomadology, but it is not essential: you can be a nomad and never travel further than your armchair. Returning from five months' study leave in which I had circumnavigated the globe, my first evening back in my home was alien, not because I was in one place, but because I could not believe that I owned this house; that there were pictures on the wall that belonged to me, and cupboards of crockery and the collected accretions of a few decades of purchases and other acquisitions. What need had I for these things? I had had all I needed in a rucksack: all these possessions made me feel heavy and ponderous, as if I was back in gravity after months in zero-G. Needless to say, this feeling wore off: though I continue to sporadically dispose of possessions.

If this were a Buddhist manifesto, the message from this little tale would be: 'let go, don't get attached to material things'. But nomadology is not saying that. Attachment is what makes us human, and we must engage with the world, not separate ourselves in some private cocoon of detachment. We must be passionate and angry, love and be loved, stand up for ourselves and for others, live and die. But our engagement – and our bodies – must always be processual, we must always be becoming, never having become. That means having a line of flight open (even if for now you choose not to take it – except that you are already on it anyway). Not being closed down by alcohol or drug dependency, gut-wrenching love affairs, sixteen-hour days at the office, fears of ageing and death or any of the other body–affect confluences which territorialize me and you into the ruts which we may even defend because that's all we see before us. That is what nomadology is about. And what is beyond health is this becoming other, the never-ending unfolding of a life of choices and chances, commission and omission, opportunities taken and missed.

I'm working on it.

Glossary

This glossary is intended to provide readers with an indication of how some terms in post-structuralism and postmodern theory are used in this book. Concepts which have a wider circulation in sociology are not included, and readers should consult a dictionary of social science terminology.

affect The emotional or other relation which a body has with other entities. For example, an alcoholic has affects with drink and with drinking.

arché-health A term coined by the author to describe a resistance to control or definition, a 'becoming-different' which is potentially emancipatory. It is not intended as any kind of prior 'health', rather it is the system of difference which makes it possible to speak of 'health' or 'illness'.

becoming A process of transformation, counterposed to a fixity of being or identity, often used to indicate a becoming 'other' or different, with no specific end-point as a goal.

Body-without-Organs (BwO) The term invented by Deleuze and Guattari (1984, 1988) to describe a non-anatomical, political body inscribed by power and desire. The BwO is the consequence of patterns of affect (q.v.) on a body.

deconstruction A strategy to explore and challenge the authority by which a statement or claim to truth or knowledge has been made.

desire Used either (in psychoanalysis) to describe the yearning to resolve a lack of some object (the object of desire), or (by Deleuze and Guattari 1984) to signify a positive investment in another person or thing.

deterritorialization See territorialization.

différance A word coined by Derrida to imply both the characteristic of language to give meaning to words in terms of their difference from other words, and the deferral of meaning as signifiers refer endlessly to others.

discourse, discursive practice Written, spoken or enacted practices organized so as to supply a coherent claim to a position or perspective. Used in post-structuralism to indicate the association between 'knowledge' and power. See also text.

essentialism, essence A philosophical perspective on human identity which locates the self as internal and existing independently and prior to social structure and/or language. Essentialism argues that the capacity to act as an individual is a consequence of this prior self.

finitude The sense of limitation in human affairs consequent upon embodiment and mortality, and the inability to experience as another.

gaze Used to describe the exercise of power through surveillance. Knowledge gained by observation is used to control the person who is the object of surveillance, and to create that person as a subject constituted through that knowledge. See also power/knowledge.

genealogy An analytical strategy which documents the ways in which a practice has been described discursively. Unlike a standard history, no effort is made to discover a rational progression of understanding of the practice, or to 'explain' why different perspectives were dominant at different points in time. Instead, discontinuities between discourses are highlighted.

gift The feminine relation of generosity and trust, opposed to the *proper* (q.v.).

haecceity An event or singularity comprising entities associated through affect (q.v.) or relationships.

intertextuality The endless reference, association or allusions which one text (q.v.) has to others. For a reader, this referentiality to further texts establishes chains of meanings for a text not necessarily intended by an author.

line of flight The 'escape route' from a territorialization (q.v.).

logocentrism The claim to authority, to be able to 'speak the truth' about something. Religion and science are logocentrisms which make particular claims to possess this authoritative knowledge.

logos Truth, or knowledge of the world or some element of it.

meta-narrative An overarching discourse or position which organizes other positions. Class and gender have been used in structuralist social theory to explain the organization of societies in terms of economics or patriarchy. Postmodernism is suspicious of any efforts to connect events or attributes within such frameworks of 'explanation', seeing meta-narratives as fabrications rather than representations of social reality.

modernity, modernism An era generally taken to have begun with the Enlightenment (*c*.1800), characterized by a philosophical commitment to the rational and/or scientific elucidation of the world, and the progressive accumulation of knowledge. Modern disciplines in the human sciences use methodological strategies to represent 'reality' more and more accurately.

nomadic subject A subjectivity freed (briefly or more extensively) from power and territorialization (q.v.), able to 'become' different, free to explore the discourses of the Body-without-Organs, to discover new possibilities for being or for action.

the Other Literally, that which is not the self: a person, thing or idea.

postmodernism Used in this book to describe a philosophical position which rejects modernist efforts to discover knowledge about the world, and replaces this with a focus upon the strategies by which such modernist knowledge-claims are made.

post-structuralism A position originally deriving from literacy theory, which rejects structuralist efforts to discover systems of meaning or meta-narratives constructed in cultural, social or political structures. The reader of a text is accorded privilege as the creator of meaning in place of the writer, whose intentions – it is concluded – can never be known decisively. In social theory, post-structuralism concerns itself with the indeterminacy in social interactions and the efforts which are made by human agents to control or define reality.

power/knowledge The linking by Foucault of power to knowledge abandons the view that power is unitary and coercive. For example, power is seen to be a consequence of expertise, a body of knowledge which is able to legitimate the rights of those who hold it to subject others to particular practices. Power is exercised in the micro-processes of interaction, in every encounter which is organized by a discourse on knowledge. It may be contested by rival discourses, based in alternative bodies of knowledge.

presence An unmediated knowledge of an aspect of the world, presence is the basis of a logocentric claim to 'know the truth'. Science claims presence – knowledge of its subject matter – through discourses on method. Presence of God is the basis of religious experience. Essentialism (q.v.) is sometimes used to make claims to presence concerning knowledge of the self, feelings or existence.

proper The masculine relation of control and possession.

reflexivity Analysis which interrogates the process by which interpretation has been fabricated: reflexivity requires any effort to describe or represent to consider how that process of description was achieved, what claims to 'presence' were made, what authority was used to claim knowledge.

reterritorialization See territorialization.

subject, subjectivity In postmodern theory, subjectivity is the outcome of power, and the subject is no more than an effect of power, constituted in discourses of power/knowledge. In this book it is argued that, in spite of this, the undecidability of meaning involved in any discursive practice enables subjectivities to be multivocal rather than fixed, and capable of 'becoming' through resistance to power/knowledge.

territorialization The process of establishing a context for a body or thing, which in the process gives it meaning. A sharpened stick is territorialized into a spear by the context of its potential to inflict or threaten harm.

text A set of signifiers – written, spoken or enacted – of which sense can be made. In this book, text is taken to include meaningful social practices.

will-to-power This term, which derives from Nietzsche, is understood as the affirmation of potential of the organism. It is the basis for the body's capacity to resist power, and to 'become-other'.

References

Adam, B. (1990) *Time and Social Theory*. Cambridge: Polity.

Adam, B. (1992) 'Time and health implicated: a conceptual critique', in Frankenberg, R. (ed.) *Time, Health and Medicine*. London: Sage.

Adam, B. (1995) *Timewatch. The Social Analysis of Time*. Cambridge: Polity.

Aiken, L. and Fagin, C. (1992) (eds) *Charting Nursing's Future*. Philadelphia: JB Lipincott.

Amos, A., Gray, D., Currie, C. and Elton, R. (1997) 'Healthy or druggy? Self-image, ideal image and smoking behaviour among young people', *Social Science & Medicine*, 45: 847–58.

Anand, P. (1993) *Foundations of Rational Choice under Risk*. Oxford: Clarendon.

Anderson, B.M. (1991) 'Mapping the terrain of the discipline', in Gray, G. and Pratt, R. (eds) *Towards a Discipline of Nursing*. Melbourne: Churchill Livingstone.

Annandale, E. and Clark, J. (1996) 'What is gender? Feminist theory and the sociology of reproduction', *Sociology of Health & Illness* 18: 17–44.

Ardener, E. (1972) 'Belief and the problem of women', in La Fontaine, J.S. (ed.) *The Interpretation of Ritual*. London: Tavistock.

Armstrong, D. (1983) *The Political Anatomy of the Body*. Cambridge: Cambridge University Press.

Armstrong, D. (1987) 'Theoretical tensions in biopsychosocial medicine', *Social Science & Medicine* 25: 1213–18.

Armstrong, D. (1994) 'Bodies of knowledge/knowledge of bodies', in Jones, C. and Porter, R. (eds) *Reassessing Foucault*. London: Routledge.

Armstrong, D. (1997) 'Foucault and the sociology of health and illness: a prismatic reading', in Petersen A. and Bunton, R. (eds) *Foucault, Health and Medicine*. London: Routledge.

Atkinson, P. (1981) *The Clinical Experience*. London: Gower.

Atkinson, P. (1990) *The Ethnographic Imagination*. London: Routledge.

Banting, P. (1992) 'The body as pictogram: rethinking Helene Cixous's *ecriture feminine*', *Textual Practices*, 25: 225–46.

Barthes, R. (1977) *Image-Music-Text*. Glasgow: Collins Fontana.

Baszanger, I. (1992) 'Deciphering chronic illness', *Sociology of Health & Illness*, 14: 181–215.

Bauman, Z. (1989) *Modernity and the Holocaust*. Cambridge: Polity.

Bauman, Z. (1993a) *Intimations of Postmodernity*. London: Routledge.

Bauman, Z. (1993b) *Postmodern Ethics*. Oxford: Blackwell.

Beck, J. and Rosenbaum, M. (1994) *Pursuit of Ecstasy: the MDMA Experience*. Albany: State University of New York Press.

Beck, U. (1992) *Risk Society*. London: Sage.

Beck, U. (1994) 'The reinvention of politics: towards a theory of reflexive modernization', in Beck, U., Giddens, A. and Lash S. (eds) *Reflexive Modernization*. Cambridge: Polity.

Benton, T. (1991) 'Biology and social science: why the return of the repressed should be given a cautious welcome', *Sociology*, 25: 1–29.

Berger, P.L. and Luckmann, T. (1971) *The Social Construction of Reality*. Harmondsworth: Penguin University Books.

Bertholet, J.M. (1991) 'Sociological discourse and the body', in Featherstone, M., Hepworth, M. and Turner, B. (eds) *The Body*. London: Sage.

Bevis, E.M. (1982) *Curriculum Building in Nursing – a Process*. St Louis: Mosby.

Biley, F. (1993) 'Ward design: creating a healing patient environment', *Nursing Standard* 8: 31–5.

Bloor, D. (1976) *Knowledge and Social Imagery*. London: Routledge.

Bloor, M. and McIntosh, J. (1990) 'Surveillance and concealment', in Cunningham-Burley, S. and McKeganey, N. *Readings in Medical Sociology*. London: Routledge.

Bocock, R. (1974) *Ritual in Industrial Society*. London: George Allen and Unwin.

Bogue, R. (1989) *Deleuze and Guattari*. London: Routledge.

Bond, J. (1991) 'The politics of care-giving: the professionalisation of informal care', paper presented to the British Sociological Association conference, Manchester.

Bourdieu, P. (1990) *In Other Words*, Cambridge: Polity Press.

Braidotti, R. (1993) 'Discontinuous becomings. Deleuze on the becoming-woman of philosophy', *Journal of the British Society for Phenomenology* 24: 44–55.

British Medical Association (1987) *Living with Risk*. Chichester: John Wiley.

Brown, B. and Cousins, M. (1986) 'The linguistic fault: the case of Foucault's archaeology', in Gane, M. (ed.) *Towards a Critique of Foucault*. London: Routledge and Kegan Paul.

Brown J.S. and Duguid, P. (1991) 'Organizational learning and communities of practice: towards a unified view of working, learning and innovation', *Organization Science* 2: 40–57.

Brubaker, R.S. (1984) *The Limits of Rationality*. London: Allen and Unwin.

Brykczynska G. (1992) 'Caring: a dying art?', in M. Jolley and G. Brykczynska G. (eds), *Nursing care: the challenge to change*. London: Edward Arnold.

Buchanan, D.R. (1991) 'How teens think about drugs: insights from moral reasoning and social bonding theory', *International Quarterly of Community Health Education* 11: 315–32.

Buchanan, I. (1997) 'The problem of the body in Deleuze and Guattari, or, what can a body do?', *Body & Society*, 3: 73–91.

Bukatman, S. (1993) 'Gibson's typewriter', in Derv, M. (ed.) *Flame Wars. The Discourse of Cyberculture*. Durham, NC: Duke University Press. (Vol. 92 (4) of the South Atlantic Quarterly.)

Bunting, S. (1993) *Rosemarie Parse. Theory of Health as Human Becoming*. Newbury Park, CA: Sage.

Butler, J. (1990) *Gender Trouble*. London: Routledge.

Cain, M. and Finch, J. (1981) 'Towards a rehabilitation of data', in Abrams, P., Deem, R., Finch, J. and Rock, P. (eds) *Practice and Progress. British Sociology 1950–80*. London: Macmillan.

Callon, M. (1986) 'Some elements of a sociology of translation: the domestication of the scallops and St Brieuac fishermen', in Law, J. (ed.) *Power, Action and Belief* (Sociological Review monograph 32). London: Routledge and Kegan Paul.

Cameron-Traub, E. (1991) 'An evolving discipline', in Gray, G. and Pratt, R. (eds) *Towards a Discipline of Nursing*. Melbourne: Churchill Livingstone.

Canguilhem, G. (1989) *The Normal and the Pathological*. New York: Zone Books.

Caputo, J.D. (1993) *Against Ethics*. Bloomington: Indiana University Press.

Carr, W. and Kemmis, S. (1986) *Becoming Critical: Knowing through Action Research.* Victoria: Deakin University Press.

Carroll, J. (1993) *Humanism. The Wreck of Western Culture.* London: Fontana.

Carter, S. (1995) 'Boundaries of danger and uncertainty: an analysis of the technological culture of risk assessment', in Gabe, J. (ed.) *Medicine, Risk and Health.* Oxford: Blackwell Publishers.

CCTA (1994) *Management of Project Risk.* Norwich: HMSO.

Charmaz, K. (1983) 'Loss of self: a fundamental form of suffering in the chronically ill', *Sociology of Health & Illness,* 5: 168–95.

Chatwin, B. (1987) *The Songlines.* London: Jonathan Cape.

Cixous, H. (1986) 'Sorties', in Cixous, H. and Clement, C. (eds) *The Newly Born Woman.* Manchester: Manchester University Press.

Cixous, H. (1990) 'The laugh of the medusa', in Walder, R. (ed.) *Literature in the Modern World.* Oxford: Oxford University Press.

Clark, J. (1993) 'Into the community', in Dolan, B. (ed.) *Project 2000: Reflection and Celebration.* London: Scutari.

Coffey, A.J. (1994) 'Timing is everything: graduate accountants, time and organisational commitment', *Sociology* 28: 943–56.

Collins, H. (1994) 'Dissecting surgery: forms of life depersonalized', *Social Studies of Science* 24: 311–33.

Cotton, N.S. and Geraty, R.G. (1984) 'Therapeutic space design : planning an in-patient children's unit', *American Journal of Orthopsychiatry,* 54: 624–36.

Counsel and Care (1993) *The Right to Take Risks.* London: Counsel and Care.

Critchley, S. (1992) *The Ethics of Deconstruction.* Oxford: Blackwell.

Cupitt, D. (1994) *After All. Religion without Alienation.* London: SCM Press.

Curt, B. (1994). *Textuality and Tectonics: Troubling Social and Psychological Science.* Buckingham: Open University Press.

Davis, A. and Horobin, G. (1977) *Medical Encounters: the Experience of Illness and Treatment.* London: Croom Helm.

Dawkins, R. (1989) *The Selfish Gene.* Oxford: Oxford University Press.

Dawson, S. (1995) 'Never mind solutions: what are the issues? Lessons of industrial technology transfer for quality in health care', *Quality in Health Care* 4: 197–203.

de Swaan, A. (1990) *The Management of Normality.* London: Routledge.

Deleuze, G. (1968) *Différance et Repetition.* Paris: PUF.

Deleuze, G. (1969, 1990) *The Logic of Sense.* New York: Columbia University Press. (French Ed.: *Logique du Sens.* Paris: Minuit).

Deleuze, G. (1988) *Foucault.* Minneapolis: University of Minnesota Press.

Deleuze, G. and Guattari, F. (1984) *Anti-Oedipus: Capitalism and Schizophrenia.* London: Athlone.

Deleuze, G. and Guattari, F. (1988) *A Thousand Plateaus.* London: Athlone.

Deleuze, G. and Guattari, F. (1994) *What is Philosophy?* London: Verso.

Department of the Environment (1995) *A Guide to Risk Assessment and Risk Management for Environmental Protection.* London: HMSO.

Derrida, J. (1976) *Of Grammatology.* Baltimore: Johns Hopkins.

Derrida, J. (1978) *Writing and Difference.* London: Routledge.

Derrida, J. (1987a) *The Post Card. From Socrates to Freud and Beyond.* Chicago: University of Chicago Press.

Derrida, J. (1987b) *The Truth in Painting.* Chicago: University of Chicago Press.

Derrida, J. (1992) *Given Time: 1. Counterfeit Money.* Chicago: University of Chicago Press.

Derrida, J. (1995) *The Gift of Death.* Chicago: University of Chicago Press.

Dolan, B. (1993) 'Reflection and celebration', in Dolan, B. (ed.) *Project 2000: Reflection and Celebration.* London: Scutari.

Donnelly, M. (1986) 'Foucault's genealogy of the human sciences', in Gane, M. (ed.) *Towards a Critique of Foucault.* London: Routledge and Kegan Paul.

Douglas, C. (1979). *Bleeders Come First.* London: Canongate.

Douglas, M. (1966) *Purity and Danger.* London: Routledge.

Douglas, M. (1992) *Risk and Blame. Essays in Cultural Theory.* London: Routledge.

Douglas, M. (1996) *Natural Symbols.* (New Edition) London: Routledge.

Dreyfus, H.L. and Rabinow, P. (1982) *Michel Foucault: Beyond Structuralism and Hermeneutics.* Chicago: University of Chicago Press.

Dunlop, M.J. (1986) 'Is a science of caring possible?', *Journal of Advanced Nursing*, 11: 661–70.

Eckermann, L. (1997) 'Foucault, embodiment and gendered subjectivities: the case of voluntary self-starvation', in Petersen A. and Bunton, R. (eds) *Foucault, Health and Medicine.* London: Routledge.

Eddy, M.B. (1994) *Science and Health.* Boston: First Church of Christ, Scientist.

Etzioni, A. (1995) *The Spirit of Community.* London: Fontana.

Flax, J. (1990). *Thinking Fragments.* Berkeley: University of California Press.

Forrester, J. (1990) *The Seductions of Psychoanalysis.* Cambridge: Cambridge University Press.

Foucault, M. (1970) *The Order of Things.* London: Tavistock.

Foucault, M. (1974) *The Archaeology of Knowledge.* London: Tavistock.

Foucault, M. (1976) *The Birth of the Clinic.* London: Tavistock.

Foucault, M. (1977a) 'What is an author?', in Bouchard, D.F. (ed.) *Language, Counter-memory, Practice.* Oxford: Blackwell.

Foucault, M. (1977b) 'History of systems of thought', in Bouchard, D.F. (ed.) *Language, Counter-memory, Practice.* Oxford: Blackwell.

Foucault, M. (1977c) 'Theatrum Philosophicum', in Bouchard, D.F. (ed.) *Language, Counter-memory, Practice.* Oxford: Blackwell.

Foucault, M. (1979) *Discipline and Punish.* Harmondsworth: Peregrine.

Foucault, M. (1980a) 'The eye of power', in Gordon, C. (ed.) *Power/Knowledge.* Brighton: Harvester.

Foucault, M. (1980b) 'Truth and power', in Gordon, C. (ed.) *Power/Knowledge.* Brighton: Harvester.

Foucault, M. (1980c) 'Two lectures', in Gordon, C. (ed.) *Power/Knowledge.* Brighton: Harvester.

Foucault, M. (1980d) 'The confession of the flesh', in Gordon, C. (ed.) *Power/Knowledge.* Brighton: Harvester.

Foucault, M. (1984) *The History of Sexuality Part 1.* Harmondsworth: Penguin.

Foucault, M. (1985) *The Use of Pleasure* (Vol. 2 of the *History of Sexuality*) New York: Pantheon.

Foucault, M. (1986) *The Care of the Self* (Vol. 3 of the *History of Sexuality*). New York: Pantheon.

Foucault, M. (1988a) 'The political technology of individuals', in Martin, L.H., Gutman, H. and Hutton, P.H. (eds) *Technologies of the Self.* London: Tavistock

Foucault, M. (1988b) 'Technologies of the self', in Martin, L.H., Gutman, H. and Hutton, P.H. (eds) *Technologies of the Self.* London: Tavistock.

Fox, N.J. (1984) 'L of a time with the advanced drivers', *In Camera,* 3: 8.

Fox, N.J. (1988) 'Scientific theory choice and social structure: the case of Lister's antisepsis, humoral theory and asepsis', *History of Science,* 26: 367–97.

Fox, N.J. (1991) 'Postmodernism, rationality and the evaluation of health care', *Sociological Review,* 39: 709–44.

Fox, N.J. (1992) *The Social Meaning of Surgery.* Buckingham: Open University Press.

Fox, N.J. (1993a) *Postmodernism, Sociology and Health.* Buckingham: Open University Press.

Fox, N.J. (1993b) 'Discourse, organization and the surgical ward round', *Sociology of Health & Illness* 15: 16–44.

Fox, N.J. (1994) 'Anaesthetists, the discourse on patient fitness and the organization of surgery', *Sociology of Health & Illness,* 16: 1–18.

Fox, N.J. (1995a) 'Postmodern perspectives on care: the vigil and the gift', *Critical Social Policy,* 15: 107–25.

Fox, N.J. (1995b) 'Professional models of school absence associated with home responsibilities', *British Journal of Sociology of Education,* 16: 221–42.

Fox, N.J. (1995c) 'Intertextuality and the writing of social research', *Electronic Journal of Sociology* 1, 3: no page numbers.

Fox, N.J. and Roberts, C. (1999) 'GPs in cyberspace: the sociology of a virtual community', *Sociological Review,* 14(4).

Fox, N.J., Dolman, E., Lane, P., O'Rourke, A. and Roberts, C. (1999) 'The WISDOM project: a virtual classroom for primary care informatics', *Medical Education,* 33: 365–70.

Freundlieb, D. (1994) 'The archaeology of Foucault', in Jones, C. and Porter, R. (eds) *Reassessing Foucault.* London; Routledge.

Game, A. (1991) *Undoing the Social.* Buckingham: Open University Press.

Gardner, K. (1992) 'The historical conflict between caring and professionalisation: a dilemma for nursing', in Gaut, D.A. (ed.), *The Presence of Caring.* New York: National League for Nursing Press.

Garfinkel, H. (1967) *Studies in Ethnomethodology.* Englewood Cliffs, NJ: Prentice Hall.

Gelsthorpe, L. (1992) 'Response to Martyn Hammersley's paper "On feminist methodology"', *Sociology,* 26, 213–18.

Giddens, A. (1984) *The Constitution of Society.* Cambridge: Polity Press.

Glassner, B. (1989) 'Fitness and the postmodern self', *Journal of Health & Social Behaviour,* 30: 180–91.

Gluckman, E. (1962) '*Les rites de passage*', in Gluckman, E. (ed.) *Essays on the Ritual of Social Relations.* Manchester: Manchester University Press.

Goffman, E. (1959) *The Presentation of Self in Everyday Life.* London: Allen Lane.

Goffman, E. (1968) *Asylums.* Harmondsworth: Penguin.

Goffman, E. (1970) *Stigma.* Harmondsworth: Penguin.

Goffman, E. (1974) *Frame Analysis: an Essay on the Organization of Experience.* New York: Harper and Row.

Goldstein, J. (1984) 'Foucault among the sociologists', *History and Theory* 15: 170–92.

Goodson, I and Dowbiggin, I. (1990) 'Docile bodies: commonalities in the history of psychiatry and schooling', in Ball, J. (ed.) *Foucault and Education.* London: Routledge.

Graham, H. (1979) 'Prevention and health: every mother's business', in Harris, C. (ed.), *The Sociology of the Family*. Keele: Keele University Press.

Graham, H. (1983) 'Caring: a labour of love', in J. Finch and D. Groves (eds), *A Labour of Love: Women, Work and Caring*. London: Routledge and Kegan Paul.

Graham, H. (1991) 'The concept of caring in feminist research', *Sociology*, 25: 61–78.

Grant, B. (1997) 'Disciplining students: the construction of student subjectivities', *British Journal of Sociology of Education*, 18: 101–14.

Gray, G. and Pratt, R. (1991) (eds) *Towards a Discipline of Nursing*. Melbourne: Churchill Livingstone.

Green, A.R. and Goodwin, G.M. (1996) 'Ecstasy and neuro-degeneration', *British Medical Journal*, 312: 1493–4.

Gregory, R. (1990) *Eye and Brain*. (4th Edition) London: Weidenfeld and Nicolson.

Grimshaw, J.M. and Russell, I.T. (1993) 'Effects of clinical guidelines on medical practice: a systematic review of rigorous evaluations', *Lancet*, 342: 1317–22.

Grinyer, A. (1995) 'Risk, the real world and naive sociology', in Gabe, J. (ed.) *Medicine, Risk and Health*. Oxford: Blackwell Publishers.

Haber, H. (1994) *Beyond Postmodern Politics. Lyotard, Rorty, Foucault*. New York: Routledge.

Hacking, I. (1986) 'The archaeology of Foucault', in Hoy, D.C. (ed.) *Foucault: a Critical Reader*. Oxford: Blackwell.

Haines, A. and Jones, R. (1994) 'Implementing findings of research', *British Medical Journal*, 308: 1488–92.

Hall, E.T. (1984) *The Dance of Life*. New York: Anchor Press.

Handy, C. (1991) 'Thinking upside down', in Henry, J. (ed.) *Creative Management*. Buckingham: Open University Press.

Haraway, D. (1991) *Simians, Cyborgs and Women*. London: Free Association Books.

Harding, J. (1997) 'Bodies at risk: sex, surveillance and hormone replacement therapy', in Petersen A. and Bunton, R. (eds) *Foucault, Health and Medicine*. London: Routledge.

Hart, E. and Bond, M. (1995) *Action Research for Health and Social Care*. Buckingham: Open University Press.

Hassler, J. (1993) 'Variations in risk – a cause of fluctuations in demand?' Seminar Paper 532. Stockholm: Institute for International Economic Studies.

Haynes, R.B. (1993) 'Some problems in applying evidence in clinical practice', *Annals of the New York Academy of Science*, 73: 21–4.

Hearn, J. and Morgan, D. (1990) *Men, Masculinities and Social Theory*. London: Unwin Hyman.

Heidegger, M. (1958) *The Question of Being*. New York: Harper and Row.

Helman, C. (1984) *Culture, Health and Illness*. Bristol: Wright.

Helman, C. (1991) *Body Myths*. London: Chatto and Windus.

Helman, C. (1992) 'Heart disease and the cultural construction of time', in Frankenberg, R. (ed.) *Time, Health and Medicine*. London: Sage.

Hertz, D.B. and Thomas, H. (1983) *Risk Analysis and its Applications*. Chichester: Wiley.

Hirschauer, S. (1991) 'The manufacture of bodies in surgery', *Social Studies of Science*, 21: 279–319.

Hochschild, A.R. (1983) *A Managed Heart*. Berkeley: University of California Press.

Holmwood, J. (1995) 'Feminism and epistemology: what kind of successor science?', *Sociology*, 29: 411–28.

Hoy, D.C. (1986) 'Introduction', in Hoy, D.C. (ed.) *Foucault: a Critical Reader.* Oxford: Blackwell.

Hughes, D. (1988) 'When nurse knows best', *Sociology of Health & Illness*, 10: 1–22.

Hugman, R. (1991) *Power in Caring Professions.* Basingstoke: Macmillan.

Hutcheon, L. (1989). *The Politics of Postmodernism.* London: Routledge.

Inglesby, E. (1992) 'Values and philosophy of nursing: the dynamic of change', in Jolley, M. and Brykczynska, G. (eds), *Nursing Care: the Challenge to Change.* London: Edward Arnold.

James, N. (1989) 'Emotional labour: skill and work in the social regulation of feelings', *Sociological Review*, 37: 15–42.

Johnstone-Bryden, I.M. (1995) *Managing Risk.* Aldershot: Avebury.

Jordan, T. (1995) 'Collective bodies: raving and the politics of Gilles Deleuze and Felix Guattari', *Body & Society*, 1: 125–44.

Kaite, B. (1988) 'The pornographer's body double: transgression is the law', in Kroker, A. and Kroker, M. (eds) *Body Invaders.* Basingstoke: Macmillan.

Katz, P. (1984). 'Ritual in the operating room', *Ethnology* 20: 335–50.

Kershaw, B. (1992) 'Nursing models', in Jolley, M. and Brykczynska, G. (eds) *Nursing Care: the Challenge to Change.* London: Edward Arnold.

Kleinman, A. (1980) *Patients and Healers in the Context of Culture.* Berkeley: University of California Press.

Kleinman, A. (1988) *The Illness Narratives.* New York: Basic Books.

Knowles, J. (1977) *Doing Better and Feeling Worse.* New York: Norton.

Kristeva, J. (1986) *The Kristeva Reader.* New York: Columbia University Press.

Kroker, A. and Kroker, M (1988) 'Panic sex in America', in Kroker A. and Kroker, M. (eds) *Body Invaders.* Basingstoke: Macmillan.

Kuhn, T. (1962) *The Structure of Scientific Revolutions.* Chicago: University of Chicago Press.

Laller, P. (1993) 'Fertile obsession: validity after post-structuralism', *Sociological Quarterly*, 34: 673–93.

Landow, G.P. (1992) *Hypertext.* Baltimore: Johns Hopkins University Press.

Lash, S. (1991) 'Genealogy and the body: Foucault/Deleuze/Nietzsche', in Featherstone, M., Hepworth, M. and Turner, B.S. (eds) *The Body.* London: Sage.

Laufman, H. (1990) 'What's happened to aseptic discipline in the OR?', *Today's OR Nurse*, 12: 15–19.

Leonard, P. (1997) *Postmodern Welfare. Reconstructing an Emancipatory Project.* London: Sage.

Levi-Strauss, C. (1986) *The Raw and the Cooked.* Harmondsworth: Penguin.

Lewin, K. (1948) *Resolving Social Conflicts.* New York: Harper and Row.

Lincoln, Y.S. and Guba, E.G. (1985) *Naturalistic Enquiry.* California: Sage.

Lupton, D. (1995) *The Imperative of Health: Public Health and the Regulated Body.* London: Sage.

Lupton, D. (1997) 'Foucault and the medicalisation critique', in Petersen, A. and Bunton, R. (eds) *Foucault, Health and Medicine.* London: Routledge.

Lynaugh, J. and Fagin, C. (1988) 'Nursing comes of age', *Image*, 20: 184–90.

Lynch, K. (1989) 'Solidary labour: its nature and marginalisation', *Sociological Review*, 37: 1–14.

Lyotard, J. (1984) *The Postmodern Condition, A Report on Knowledge.* Minneapolis: University of Minnesota Press.

Lyotard, J. (1988) *The Differend: Phrases in Dispute.* Minneapolis: University of Minnesota Press.

Maines, D.R. (1993). 'Narrative's moment and sociology's phenomena: towards a narrative sociology', *Sociological Quarterly*, 34: 17–38.

Malin, N. and Teasdale K. (1991) 'Caring versus empowerment: considerations for nursing practice', *Journal of Advanced Nursing*, 16: 657–62.

Marsden, D. and Abrams, S. (1987) ' "Allies", "Liberators", "Intruders" and "Cuckoos in the Nest": a sociology of caring relationships over the life cycle', in Allatt, P. *et al.* (eds) *Women and the Life Cycle.* London: Macmillan.

Martin, R. (1988) 'Truth, power, self: an interview with Michel Foucault', in Martin, L.H., Gutman, H. and Hutton, P.H. (eds) *Technologies of the Self.* London: Tavistock.

Maseide, P. (1991) 'Possibly abusive, often benign, and always necessary. On power and domination in medical practice', *Sociology of Health & Illness*, 13: 545–61.

Maslow, A.H. (1968) *Towards a Psychology of Being.* New York: Van Nostrand Reinhold.

Massumi, B. (1992) *A Users' Guide to Capitalism and Schizophrenia.* Cambridge, Mass.: MIT Press.

Mauss, M. (1990) *The Gift: the Form and Reason for Exchange in Archaic Societies.* London: Routledge.

Mauthner, N.S., Parry, O. and Backett-Milburn, K. (1998) 'The data are out there, or are they? Implications for archiving and revisiting qualitative data', *Sociology*, 32: 733–45.

Mayall, B. and Foster, M. C. (1989) *Child Health Care.* Oxford: Heinemann.

McNay, L. (1992) *Foucault and Feminism.* Oxford: Polity.

Miles, A. (1991) *Women, Health and Medicine.* Buckingham: Open University Press.

Mitchell, J.C. (1983) 'Case and situation analysis', *Sociological Review*, 31: 187–211.

Mitchell, S. (1991) *The Gospel According to Jesus.* New York: HarperCollins.

Moi, T. (1985) *Sexual Textual Politics.* London: Methuen.

Moore, S.D. (1994) *Post-structuralism and the New Testament: Foucault and Derrida at the Foot of the Cross.* Minneapolis: Fortress Press.

Morgan, G. (1997) *Images of Organisation.* London: Sage.

Mouzelis, N. (1995) *Sociological Theory: What Went Wrong.* London: Routledge.

Mulkay, M.J. (1985) *The Word and the World.* London: George Allen and Unwin.

Nettleton, S. (1992) *Power, Pain and Dentistry.* Buckingham: Open University Press.

Nettleton, S. (1995) *The Sociology of Health and Illness.* Oxford: Polity.

Nixon, J. (1981) *A Teacher's Guide to Action Research.* London: Grant McIntyre.

Oakley, A. (1998) 'Gender, methodology and people's ways of knowing: some problems with feminism and the paradigm debate in social science,' *Sociology*, 32: 707–31.

Ostrander, G. (1988) 'Foucault's disappearing body', in Kroker A. and Kroker, M. (eds) *Body Invaders.* Basingstoke: Macmillan.

Owen, D. (1997) 'The postmodern challenge to sociology', in Owen, D. (ed.) *Sociology After Postmodernism.* London: Sage.

Paden, W.E. (1988) 'Theaters of humility and suspicion: desert saints and New England puritans', in Martin, L.H., Gutman, H. and Hutton, P.H. (eds) *Technologies of the Self.* London: Tavistock.

Parse, R. (1987) *Nursing Science: Major Paradigms, Theories and Critiques.* Philadelphia: WB Saunders.

Parse, R., Coyne, A.B. and Smith, M.J. (1985) *Nursing Research: Qualitative Methods.* Bowie, Maryland: Brady.

Parsons, T. (1951) *The Social System.* New York: Free Press.

Parsons, T. and Fox, R. (1952) 'Illness, therapy and the modern American family', *Journal of Social Issues,* 8: 31–44.

Patton, P. (1995) 'Mabo, freedom and the politics of difference', *Australian Journal of Political Science,* 30: 108–19.

Perakyla, A. (1989) 'Appeals to the experience of the patient in the case of dying', *Sociology of Health and Illness,* 11: 117–34.

Petersen, A. (1997) 'Risk, governance and the new public health', in Petersen A. and Bunton, R. (eds) *Foucault, Health and Medicine.* London: Routledge.

Pfohl, F. and Gordon, A. (1988) 'Criminological displacements', in Kroker A. and Kroker, M. (eds) *Body Invaders.* Basingstoke: Macmillan.

Pizzorno, A. (1992) 'Foucault and the liberal view of the individual', in Armstrong, T.J. (ed.) *Michel Foucault, Philosopher.* New York: Harvester Wheatsheaf.

Plant, S. (1993) 'Nomads and revolutionaries', *Journal of the British Society for Phenomenology,* 24: 88–101.

Poster, M. (1986) 'Foucault and the tyranny of Greece', in Hoy, D.C. (ed.) *Foucault: a Critical Reader.* Oxford: Blackwell.

Power, R., Power, T. and Gibson, N. (1996) 'Attitudes and experiences of drug use amongst a group of London teenagers', *Drugs: Education Prevention and Policy,* 3: 71–80.

Prior, L. (1987) 'Policing the dead: a sociology of the mortuary', *Sociology,* 21: 355–76.

Prior, L. (1988) 'The architecture of the hospital', *British Journal of Sociology,* 39: 86–113.

Prior, L. (1995) 'Chance and modernity: accidents as a public health problem', in Bunton, R., Nettleton, S. and Burrows, R. (eds) *The Sociology of Health Promotion.* London: Routledge.

Probyn, E. (1988) 'The anorexic body', in Kroker A. and Kroker, M. (eds) *Body Invaders.* Basingstoke: Macmillan.

Radley, A. (1989) 'Style, discourse and constraints in adjustment to chronic illness', *Sociology of Health & Illness,* 11: 230–52.

Ramazanoglu, C. (1992) 'On feminist methodology: male reason versus female empowerment', *Sociology,* 26, 207–12.

Rawlings, B. (1989) 'Coming clean: the symbolic use of clinical hygiene in a hospital sterilising unit', *Sociology of Health & Illness,* 11: 279–93.

Rayner, S. (1992) 'Cultural theory and risk analysis', in Krimsky, S. and Golding, D. (eds) *Social Theories of Risk.* Westport, Co: Praeger.

Reinharz, S. (1984) *On Becoming a Social Scientist.* New Brunswick, NJ: Transaction Books.

Riehl, J.P. and Roy, C. (1980) (eds) *Conceptual Models for Nursing Practice.* New York: Appleton Century Crofts.

Roberts, H. (1985) *The Patient Patients.* London: Routledge and Kegan Paul.

Rogers, R. and Salvage, J. (1988) *Nurses at Risk. A Guide to Health and Safety at Work.* London: Heinemann.

Rorty, R. (1992) 'Moral identity and private autonomy', in Armstrong, T.J. (ed.) *Michel Foucault, Philosopher.* New York: Harvester Wheatsheaf.

Rose, N. (1989) *Governing the Soul.* London: Routledge.

Rosenau, P.M. (1992) *Postmodernism and the Social Sciences*. Princeton, NJ: Princeton University Press.

Rosengren, W.R. and DeVault, S. (1963) 'The sociology of time and space in an obstetrical hospital', in Freidson, E. (ed.) *The Hospital in Modern Society*. New York: Free Press.

Roth, J. (1963) *Timetables*. Indianapolis: Bobbs Merrill.

Rushkoff, R. (1994) *Cyberia*. Glasgow: HarperCollins.

Sackett, D.L., Rosenberg, M.C., Muir Gray, J.A., Haynes, R.B. and Scott Richardson, W. (1996) 'Evidence-based medicine; what it is and what it isn't', *British Medical Journal*, 12: 71–2.

Sacks, O. (1991) *Awakenings*. London: Picador.

Sacks, O. (1995) *An Anthropologist on Mars: Seven Paradoxical Tales*. London: Picador.

Salvage, J. (1989) 'Selling ourselves', *Nursing Times*, 85: 24.

Saunders, N. (1995) 'The Leah Betts Story', published at WWW address: http://obsolete.org/index.html

Sawicki, J. (1991) *Disciplining Foucault: Feminism, Power and the Body*. New York: Routledge.

Scambler, G. and Hopkins, A. (1986) 'Being epileptic: coming to terms with stigma', *Sociology of Health & Illness*, 8: 26–43.

Schensul, J.J. (1987) 'Perspectives on collaborative research', in Stull, D.D. and Schensul, J.J. (eds) *Collaborative Research and Social Change*. Boulder, Co: Westview Press.

Schensul, J.J., Dennelli-Hess, D., Borrero, M.G. and Bhavati, M-P. (1987) 'Urban Comadromes: maternal and child health research and policy formulation in a Puerto-Rican community', in Stull, D.D. and Schensul, J.J. (eds) *Collaborative Research and Social Change*. Boulder, Co: Westview Press.

Sedgewick, P. (1982) *Psychopolitics*. London: Pluto Press.

Sewell, G. and Wilkinson, B. (1992) ' "Someone to watch over me": surveillance, discipline and the Just-in-Time labour process', *Sociology*, 26: 271–90.

Shaugnessy, A.F., Slanson, D.C. and Bennett, J.H. (1994) 'Becoming an information master: a guidebook to the medical information jungle', *Journal of Family Practice*, 39: 89–99.

Shrock, R.A. (1982) 'Is health visiting a profession?', *Health Visitor*, 55: 104–6.

Shutz, A. (1962) *Concepts and Theory Formation in the Social Sciences (Collected Papers Vol. 1)*. Copenhagen: Martinus Nijhoff.

Silverman, D. (1983) 'The clinical subject: adolescents in a cleft palate clinic', *Sociology of Health and Illness*, 5: 253–74.

Silverman, D. (1985) *Qualitative Methodology and Sociology*. Aldershot: Gower.

Sims, S. (1991) 'The nature and relevance of theory for practice', in Gray, G. and Pratt, R. (eds) *Towards a Discipline of Nursing*. Melbourne: Churchill Livingstone.

Smart, B. (1985) *Michel Foucault*. London: Tavistock.

Stacey, M. (1988) *The Sociology of Health and Healing*. London: Unwin Hyman.

Stanley, L. and Morgan, D. (1993). 'Editorial introduction', *Sociology*. 27: 1–4.

Starkey, K. (1992) 'Time and the hospital consultant', in Frankenberg, R. (ed.) *Time, Health and Medicine*. London: Sage.

Stonach, I. and MacLure, M. (1997) *Educational Research Undone: the Postmodern Embrace*. Buckingham: Open University Press.

Stone, A.R. (1992) 'Will the real body stand up? Boundary stories about virtual cultures', in Benedikt, M. (ed.) *Cyberspace. First Steps*. Cambridge, Mass.: MIT Press.

Strauss, A., Fagerhaugh, S., Suczek, B. and Wiener, C. (1985) *Social Organization of Medical Work*. Chicago: University of Chicago Press.

Strong, P. (1978) *The Ceremonial Order of the Clinic*. London: Routledge.

Strumpf, N.E. and Stevenson, C.M. (1992) 'Breaking new ground in elder care: practice, research and education', in Aiken, L. and Fagin, C. (1992) (eds) *Charting Nursing's Future*. Philadelphia: JB Lippincott.

Stull, D.D. and Schensul, J.J. (1987) (eds) *Collaborative Research and Social Change*. Boulder, Co: Westview Press.

Summers, A. (1979) 'Home from home: women's philanthropic work in the nineteenth century', in Burman, S. (ed.) *Fit Work for Women*. London: Croom Helm.

Suter, G.W. (1993) *Ecological Risk Assessment*. Chelsea, MI: Lewis Publishers.

Thomas, C. (1993) 'Deconstructing concepts of care', *Sociology*, 27: 649–70.

Thomas, J. and Dolan, B. (1993) 'The changing face of nursing: 2000 and beyond', in Dolan, B. (ed.) *Project 2000: Reflection and Celebration*. London: Scutari.

Thorogood, N. (1995) ' "London dentist in HIV scare": HIV and dentistry in popular discourse', in Bunton, R., Nettleton, S. and Burrows, R. (eds) *The Sociology of Health Promotion*. London: Routledge.

Trites, D.K., Galbraith, F.D., Sturdavant, M. and Leckwart, J.F. (1970) 'Influences of Nursing-Unit design on the activities and subjective feelings of nursing personnel', *Environment and Behaviour*, 2: 303–34.

Tuckett, D., Boulton, M., Olson, C. and Williams, A. (1985) *Meetings between Experts*. London: Tavistock.

Turner, B. (1992) *Regulating Bodies*. London: Routledge.

Turner, V. (1968) *The Drums of Affliction*. Oxford: Clarendon Press.

Twinn, S.F. (1991) 'Conflicting paradigms of health visiting: a continuing debate for professional practice', *Journal of Advanced Nursing*, 16: 966–73.

Tyler, D. (1997) 'At risk of maladjustment: the problem of child mental health', in Petersen, A. and Bunton, R. (eds) *Foucault, Health and Medicine*. London: Routledge.

Tyler, S.A. (1986). 'Postmodern ethnography', in Clifford, J. and Marcus, G.E. (eds) *Writing Culture: the Poetics and Politics of Ethnography*. Berkeley: University of California Press.

Ungerson, C. (1987) *Policy is Personal: Sex, Gender and Informal Care*. London: Tavistock.

van Leeuwen, C.J. (1995) 'General introduction', in van Leeuwen, C.J. and Hermes, J.L.M. (eds) *Risk Assessment of Chemicals*. Dordrecht: Kluwer Academic Publishers.

Watson, H., Wood-Harper, T. and Wood, B. (1995) 'Interpreting methodology under erasure: between theory and practice', *Systems Practice*, 8: 441–68.

Weber, M. (1971) *The Protestant Ethic and the Spirit of Capitalism*. London: Unwin University Books.

Weedon, C. (1987) *Feminist Practice and Post-structuralist Theory*. Oxford: Basil Blackwell.

Wells, G.L. (1996) *Hazard Identification and Risk Assessment*. Rugby: Institute of Chemical Engineers.

White S. (1991) *Political Theory and Postmodernism*. Cambridge: Cambridge University Press.

WHO (1985) *Targets for Health for All*. Geneva: World Health Organisation.

Wickham, G. (1986) 'Power and power analysis: beyond Foucault?', in Gane, M. (ed.) *Towards a Critique of Foucault.* London: Routledge.

Williams, S. and Bendelow, G. (1998) 'Emotions in social life: mapping the socio-logical terrain', in Bendelow, G. and Williams, S. (eds) *Emotions in Social Life. Critical Themes and Contemporary Issues.* London: Routledge.

Williamson, P. (1992) 'From dissemination to use: management and organisational barriers to the application of health services research findings', *Health Bulletin,* 50: 8–86.

Winter, R. (1989) *Learning From Experience.* London: Falmer Press.

Wood, M., Ferlie, E. and Fitzgerald, L. (1998) 'Achieving clinical behaviour change: a case of becoming indeterminate', *Social Science & Medicine,* 47: 1729–38.

Woolgar, S. (1988) *Science: The Very Idea.* Chichester: Ellis Horwood.

Wright W. (1982) *The Social Logic of Health.* New Brunswick: Rutgers University Press.

Wynne, B. (1992) 'Risk and social learning: reification to engagement', in Krimsky, S. and Golding, D. (eds) *Social Theories of Risk.* Westport, Co: Praeger.

Zerubavel, I. (1979) *Patterns of Time in Hospital Life.* Chicago: Chicago University Press.

Zuber-Skerritt, O. (1991) *Action Research in Higher Education.* Brisbane: Centre for Advancement of Learning and Teaching.

Author Index

233

Subject Index